Increasing knowledge of the neuroscientific basis of higher cortical integration, together with evidence from brain imaging and post-mortem studies, has in recent years led to growing recognition that abnormal brain morphology and physiology are essential components of schizophrenia. This volume was planned in order to review the neurodevelopmental processes and mechanisms that may be involved in the etiology and expression of schizophrenia. In particular, it sets out to examine the evidence pointing to a role for prenatal and perinatal events in the origins of the brain anomalies which may underlie the condition.

In this context, contributors review the normal development of the human brain, the ways in which fetal neural developmental anomalies and delivery complications may produce a damaged infant brain, and how such defects may predispose to schizophrenia.

By attempting to explain the complex syndromes of adult schizophrenia in terms of fetal developmental anomalies, this volume reexamines much basic information on human brain growth and how that growth may be best protected. It is an essential contribution to the debate on the etiology of schizophrenia, and as such will be of interest to all neuroscientists and psychiatric investigators.

FETAL NEURAL DEVELOPMENT AND ADULT SCHIZOPHRENIA

LONGITUDINAL PERSPECTIVES
IN SCHIZOPHRENIA RESEARCH

FETAL NEURAL DEVELOPMENT AND ADULT SCHIZOPHRENIA

EDITED BY

SARNOFF A. MEDNICK

TYRONE D. CANNON

CHRISTOPHER E. BARR

AND **MELVIN LYON**

*Department of Psychology
and Social Science Research Institute
University of Southern California*

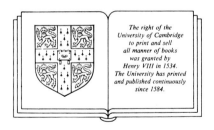

*The right of the
University of Cambridge
to print and sell
all manner of books
was granted by
Henry VIII in 1534.
The University has printed
and published continuously
since 1584.*

CAMBRIDGE UNIVERSITY PRESS

CAMBRIDGE

NEW YORK   PORT CHESTER

MELBOURNE   SYDNEY

Published by the Press Syndicate of the University of Cambridge
The Pitt Building, Trumpington Street, Cambridge CB2 IRP
40 West 20th Street, New York, NY 10011-4211, USA
10 Stamford Road, Oakleigh, Victoria 3166, Australia

First published 1991

Printed in Great Britain at the University Press, Cambridge

British Library cataloguing in publication data
Fetal neural development and adult schizophrenia.
1. Schizophrenia
I. Mednick, Sarnoff A. (Sarnoff Andrei)
616 .8982

Library of Congress cataloguing in publication data
Fetal neural development and adult schizophrenia / edited by
Sarnoff A. Mednick . . . [et al.].
p. cm.
Includes bibliographical references and index.
ISBN 0-521-39158-X (hardcover)
1. Schizophrenia – Etiology 2. Fetal brain – Abnormalities –
Consequences and sequelae. 3. Brain – Growth. I. Mednick, Sarnoff A.
[DNLM: 1. Brain – abnormalities. 2. Brain – embryology.
3. Pregnancy Complications. 4. Schizophrenia – etiology.
5. Schizophrenia – genetics. 6. Schizophrenia – pathology. WM 203 F419]
RC514.F44 1991
616.89'82071 – dc20 91-13539 CIP

ISBN 0 521 39158 X hardback

Contents

Contributors

CHRISTOPHER E. BARR, MA, University of Southern California, Social Science Research Institute, University Park, Los Angeles, California 90089-1111, USA.

BERNHARD BOGERTS, MD, University of Düsseldorf, Department of Psychiatry, Postfach 12 05 10, D-4000 Düsseldorf 12, Federal Republic of Germany.

NANCY A. BRESLIN, MD, Clinical Brain Disorders Branch, Intramural Research Program, National Institute of Mental Health, Neuroscience Research Center, 2700 Martin Luther King, Jr. Avenue, SE, Washington, DC 20032, USA.

TYRONE D. CANNON, PhD, University of Southern California, Social Science Research Institute, University Park, Los Angeles, California 90089-1111, USA.

JEFFREY A. COFFMAN, MD, Department of Psychiatry, The Ohio State University College of Medicine, 473 West 12th Avenue, Columbus, Ohio 43210, USA.

EDWARD G. JONES, MD, PhD, Department of Anatomy and Neurobiology, 317 Medical Surgery II, University of California, Irvine, California 92717, USA.

MELVIN LYON, PhD, University of Southern California, Social Science Research Institute, University Park, Los Angeles, California 90089-1111, USA.

SARNOFF A. MEDNICK, PhD, DrMed, University of Southern

ix

California, Social Science Research Institute, University Park, Los Angeles, California 90089-1111, USA.

KJELD MØLLGÅRD, MD, Embryology–Neurobiology Section, Medical Anatomy A and Center for Neuroscience, The Panum Institute, University of Copenhagen, Blegdamsvej 3, DK-2200 Copenhagen N, Denmark.

TORBEN MOOS, MD, Embryology–Neurobiology Section, Medical Anatomy A and Center for Neuroscience, The Panum Institute, University of Copenhagen, Blegdamsvej 3, DK-2200 Copenhagen N, Denmark.

HENRY A. NASRALLAH, MD, Department of Psychiatry, The Ohio State University College of Medicine, 473 West 12th Avenue, Columbus, Ohio 43210, USA.

RICHARD S. NOWAKOWSKI, PhD, Department of Neuroscience and Cell Biology, University of Medicine and Dentistry of New Jersey, Robert Wood Johnson Medical School, 675 Hoes Lane, Piscataway, New Jersey 08854, USA.

STEPHEN C. OLSON, MD, Department of Psychiatry, The Ohio State University College of Medicine, 473 West 12th Avenue, Columbus, Ohio 43210, USA.

STEVEN B. SCHWARZKOPF, MD, Department of Psychiatry, The Ohio State University College of Medicine, 473 West 12th Avenue, Columbus, Ohio 43210, USA.

METTE STAGAARD, MD, Embryology–Neurobiology Section, Medical Anatomy A and Center for Neuroscience, The Panum Institute, University of Copenhagen, Blegdamsvej 3, DK-2200 Copenhagen N, Denmark.

DANIEL R. WEINBERGER, MD, Clinical Brain Disorders Branch, Intramural Research Program, National Institute of Mental Health, Neuroscience Research Center, 2700 Martin Luther King, Jr. Avenue, SE, Washington, DC 20032, USA.

Acknowledgements

This volume reports the proceedings of a meeting on Fetal Neural Development held in Washington, DC, 30 May–1 June, 1988. We thank the National Institute of-Mental Health for help with the administrative aspects of the progam and for funding. NIMH must be commended for committing resources to this type of scientific activity.

Mednick's work on this volume was supported by NIMH grants MH 00619 (Research Scientist Award), MH 46014, MH 41469, MH 44188, MH 37692 and NARSAD, National Alliance for Research on Schizophrenia.

Cannon's work on this volume was supported by an NIMH Fellowship MH 09929 and a fellowship from the Scottish Rite Schizophrenia Research Program.

The production of the volume was also assisted by the staff and facilities of the Social Science Research Institute (Ward Edwards, Director), University of Southern California.

Part I

Introduction

1

Fetal development, birth and the syndromes of adult schizophrenia

SARNOFF A. MEDNICK AND TYRONE D. CANNON

University of Southern California

Introduction

The year 1989 saw the 50th anniversary of what was apparently the first empirical test of the hypothesis that obstetrical factors are important in the etiology of schizophrenia. In June 1939, the Faculty of the University of Southern California approved a dissertation by Barney Katz entitled 'The etiology of the deteriorating psychoses of adolescence and early adult life'. Over a $2\frac{1}{2}$-year period, Barney Katz gathered hospital obstetrical data on 100 male schizophrenics and 100 male controls. The results of his study supported the hypothesis that obstetrical factors play a role in the etiology of schizophrenia. Barney Katz's hypothesis was first suggested by his advisor, Aaron Rosanoff, who was responsible for so many innovative studies and theories in psychiatry.

Recently developed lines of evidence suggest that Rosanoff's hypothesis deserves continued study.

Neuropathology studies

Bogerts, Meertz & Schonfeldt-Bausch (1985), Jakob & Beckmann (1986), and Kovelman & Scheibel (1984) have conducted post-mortem studies of the brains of schizophrenics and have reported neuropathological deviance which they interpret as resulting from disruption of fetal neural development during the second trimester of gestation.

3

Obstetrical complications

In a recent review, McNeil (1988) concludes that schizophrenics tend to experience elevated levels of pre- and perinatal complications. There is now very good reason to believe that these obstetrical complications result in brain damage which is later reflected in the deficits noted in brain imaging studies of adult schizophrenics (see Chapter 9).

In our own research we have noted that increased ventricle–brain ratios and third ventricle widths in adulthood are significantly related to evidence of perinatal complications recorded by midwives who attended the deliveries (Silverton et al., 1985; Cannon, Mednick & Parnas, 1989). It should be noted that in these studies there were 33 years between the midwife's observation of the birth and the adult measurement of the ventricles.

Minor physical anomalies

Minor physical anomalies are benign congenital abnormalities associated with disruptions of fetal development. These external signs have been used as indices of cryptic fetal neural developmental anomalies produced by genetic factors and/or teratogens. Several investigators have reported a significantly increased frequency of these anomalies in schizophrenics (see Chapter 6).

Second trimester virus exposure

In the context of a Helsinki birth cohort exposed to a severe Type A2 influenza epidemic, we examined the hypothesis that exposure to viral infection during fetal neural development may increase risk for schizophrenia. Examination of psychiatric hospital records, when the subjects were aged 26, revealed that rates of adult schizophrenia were elevated for those exposed to the epidemic during their second trimester of fetal development. First- or third-trimester exposure was not associated with an elevation. The finding is reliable; it held independently for males and females and separately in each of several of the psychiatric hospitals in the Helsinki area (Mednick et al., 1988). We recently made another sweep of the Helsinki mental hospital records; the subjects were then 29.7 years of age. The results of the analysis of the data from this sweep were identical to those in the previous report (Machon et al., 1990). One interpretation of these results implicates a

4

disturbance in fetal neural development in the second trimester as a factor increasing the risk for adult schizophrenia.

Barr, Mednick & Munk-Jorgensen (1990) have examined 40 years of influenza and schizophrenia data from Denmark (1910–1950). For each month over those 40 years, we determined the number of live births for Denmark, the number of those born who were eventually diagnosed schizophrenic, and the number of cases of influenza reported to the Danish Ministry of Health. This study included over 7500 schizophrenics, which permitted an analysis of the possible effect of the influenza in each month of fetal development. Unusually high levels of influenza occurring during the sixth month of fetal development (and only the sixth month!) are related to unusually high levels of births of individuals who later became adult schizophrenics.

Purpose of volume

These observations suggest the hypothesis that obstetrical events play a role in the etiology of schizophrenia. This general hypothesis forms the basis of this volume. More specifically, this volume considers: (1) the normal development of the fetal brain (see Chapters 2 and 3); (2) ways in which fetal neural developmental anomalies and complications of delivery may produce a less than perfectly developed, and/or damaged, infant brain (see Chapters 4–8); (3) how such brain defects may predispose the affected individual to disordered mental functioning and behavioral deviance leading to the specific symptoms of adult schizophrenia (see Chapters 9–11). Hypothesizing a causal link between perinatal events and adult schizophrenia (with an onset 20–30 years later) may seem a hazardous enterprise. Therefore an illustrative explanation of how such a link might develop may have heuristic value. In this chapter, we present an attempt at such an explanation drawn from a theory which we favor; we also relate empirical support for these ideas from our research in Scandinavia.

The Copenhagen high-risk study: antecedents of schizophrenia

Genetic factors

In our 1962 Copenhagen high-risk study, all of the 15 schizophrenics ascertained in 1972 had schizophrenic mothers. Most also had schizophrenia spectrum fathers (Parnas, 1985). Those with schizophrenic mothers and spectrum fathers are considered to be at 'super-high risk' for schizophrenia (Gottesman & Shields, 1982). These findings mirror the robustness of the finding that some genetically transmitted factor(s) predispose to schizophrenia.

Delivery complications

Another early antecedent of adult schizophrenia among the high-risk subjects was severe delivery complications (Parnas *et al.*, 1982). It is significant that seemingly identical delivery complications among the low-risk subjects were not associated with schizophrenia. It is also significant that the delivery complications were especially strongly related to schizophrenia and ventriculomegaly among the super-high risk individuals. In other words, the greater the genetic risk (super-high risk > high risk > low risk) the stronger the relationship between delivery complications and schizophrenia and ventriculomegaly (Cannon *et al.*, 1989; 1990a,b). A part of the expression of the genetic predisposition seems to render the affected fetal brain especially vulnerable to birth trauma. This suggests that: (1) the phenotypic expression of the genetic predisposition for schizophrenia is already expressed at some time prior to delivery; and (2) the phenotypic expression of the genetic predisposition takes the form of a fragile brain, which is especially vulnerable to injury by delivery complications.

The two-hit hypothesis

The first hit: genetics

Based on these observations, we hypothesize that an important part of the phenotypic expression of the genetic predisposition to schizophrenia consists of disruptions in fetal neural development, especially in the migration, positioning and connecting of young neurons (see Chapters 2 and 3). Fetal neural disruption may also be induced by teratogenic events (e.g. a viral infection) occurring during 'schizophrenia-critical' periods of gestation. During 'schizophrenia-critical' periods, such teratogens may partially mimic or augment an existing genetically-based developmental disruption.

Our epidemiological findings (i.e. Helsinki and Denmark influenza virus studies) suggest that, for schizophrenics, the critical period during gestation occurs at some time during the second trimester. What is characteristic of brain development during this period? Brain growth exhibits maximal acceleration towards the end of the second trimester.

By the fifth month of gestation almost all of the neurons slated to comprise the human neocortex have been generated but many have not yet migrated to their target structures and become positioned and synaptically connected. The corpus callosum and vermis of the cerebellum only begin to develop or proliferate during the fourth month. Early in the second trimester the mesolimbic system (hippocampus, nucleus accumbens, ventral tegmental area, amygdala, septal region), the thalamus and the entorhinal region are experiencing rapid growth. These processes are complex and must be completed with precision. Disturbances occurring during active development of a brain area may produce incomplete or inappropriate migration, incorrect positioning, failures of connection and/or misconnections (see Chapters 2–4).

The symptoms of the schizophrenia-spectrum

We suggest that disorderly brain development during gestation is responsible for some fundamental aspects of the symptomatology of the schizophrenia-spectrum such as disorderly thought processes, eccentricity, sensory–motor coordination difficulty, and poor autonomic nervous system regulation. The genetically-programmed fetal neural disruption is considered to be responsible for the basic symptoms of all forms of the schizophrenia-spectrum. If infants with the genetically-based neural developmental anomalies have a complication-free delivery and if their social and family networks are supportive and they are protected from excessive stress in childhood and early adolescence, they will escape schizophrenia. Their cognitive, coordination and autonomic symptoms, however, may tend to increase their risk of being diagnosed schizotypal personality disorder. Schizotypal personality disorder is conceived as the basic genetic disorder; schizophrenia-proper is a complication brought on by unfortunate post-gestational experiences such as obstetrical complications and unfortunate child-rearing circumstances. We suggest that the 'first hit' increasing the risk for schizophrenia consists of the failure of normal brain development during the second trimester.

The second hit: environmental determinants

The level and type of stress imposed by the post-gestational environment may help to determine risk of decompensation and the specific course of schizophrenia. We propose, more specifically, that the circumstances of birth and early family and school–social experience of those with the

7

genetic–gestational disturbance is important in determining their risk for schizophrenic breakdown and the type of symptom-pattern and the course of their illness (Cannon et al., 1990a,b). We will discuss two types of course of illness: patients exhibiting predominantly negative symptoms and patients exhibiting predominantly positive symptoms.

We readily acknowledge that almost all schizophrenics evidence some aspects of both negative and positive symptoms in the course of their illness. When we classify a schizophrenic as a predominantly negative-symptom schizophrenic, we refer to an individual who, at an early stage of illness, may have occasionally reported a vague delusion or auditory hallucination, but whose symptom picture was dominated by anhedonia, anergia, etc. This early symptom pattern will not change markedly over the course of the illness. A predominantly positive-symptom schizophrenic at an early stage of illness will evidence anhedonia and social avoidance, but these symptoms will be overshadowed by a florid pattern of delusions, hallucinations and thought disorder. Over the course of the illness this pattern may change for some schizophrenics; the negative symptoms may become increasingly dominant.

The second hit: A. Delivery complications

A fetus with these second-trimester developmental handicaps then faces birth. It has been noted that a significantly elevated proportion of schizo-phrenics experience a difficult delivery (McNeil, 1988). Delivery difficulties are associated with indices of structural brain anomalies noted in adult schizophrenics, including significant widening of the third and lateral ventricles (see Chapter 9). In the Copenhagen high-risk project we have noted a marked interaction effect; those with especially high genetic risk for schizophrenia who also experience delivery complications evidence severe widening of the ventricles (Cannon et al., 1989). Perhaps genetically-based neural structural and vascular anomalies during gestation give rise to the special vulnerability of these high-risk fetuses to delivery difficulties.

What are the consequences for high-risk infants of these widened ventricles, which are apparently (at least in part) the sequelae of delivery complications? Several important excitatory centers of the autonomic nervous system, including the anterior hypothalamus, are located on or near the third ventricle (Darrow, 1937; Larsen, Schneiderman & Pasin, 1986; Venables & Christie, 1973; Wang, 1964). Damage to the tissue surrounding the third ventricle is likely to injure the anterior hypothalamus, which is the most important excitatory center of the autonomic nervous system. We hypothesized, therefore, that extensive damage to the periventricular tissue of the third ventricle would significantly reduce autonomic nervous system responsiveness. In support of this hypothesis, Cannon *et al.* (1988) report that, in the Copenhagen high-risk sample, widened third ventricles are significantly associated with severely reduced autonomic nervous system responsiveness in both skin conductance and heart rate. Schizophrenics with severely reduced autonomic nervous system responsiveness have been identified in the literature as autonomic nonresponders; they tend to be schizophrenics with predominantly negative symptoms (Bartfai *et al.*, 1987 and 1983; Frith *et al.*, 1979). In the Copenhagen high-risk project, non-responding schizophrenics also tend to evidence predominantly negative symptoms (Cannon *et al.*, 1990b). Thus, those with genetically-determined disruption of fetal brain development (with attendant cognitive, motor and sensory disturbances), who also suffer severe damage to excitatory autonomic nervous system areas due to delivery complications, may have a reduced capacity for emotional expressiveness and an increased risk of predominantly negative-symptom schizophrenia.

These statements are illustrated in Fig. 1.1 in the form of a decision-tree analysis. There were 138 high-risk subjects for whom complete data were available for all the variables in Fig. 1.1. The rate of predominantly negative-symptom schizophrenia in the high-risk sample is 4%. If the individual is at super-high risk (i.e. has a spectrum father) the rate of negative-symptom schizophrenia increases to 11%. If the individual has experienced above-average delivery complications then the rate of negative-symptom schizo-phrenia is 35%. If (in 1962) these individuals were also autonomic nervous system nonresponders, the rate of negative-symptom schizophrenia is 86%! Note that 130 of 131 high-risk subjects (including eight schizophrenics with dominant positive symptoms) are classified by this model as NOT having negative-symptom schizophrenia. Only one of these 131 cases is misclassified.

We hypothesize that individuals who experience the first (genetic) hit and the second (delivery complications) hit are at very high risk for predomi-nantly negative-symptom schizophrenia.

The second hit: B. Disruption of the early family rearing environment

As mentioned above, the schizophrenics in the Copenhagen high-risk study evidenced a significantly elevated level of delivery complications. The delivery complication scores for the schizophrenics had a very large variance. Accordingly, we noted that many of the high-risk subjects who became schizophrenic had experienced no delivery difficulties; such individuals had narrow third ventricles and tended to be autonomically hyperresponsive in adolescence (Cannon *et al.*, 1988, 1990a).

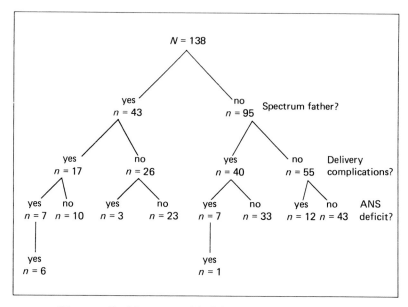

Figure 1.1 Decision-tree model of the etiology of
predominantly negative-symptom schizophrenia in the high-risk
group. Spectrum father indicates schizophrenia-spectrum
illness in the father. ANS indicates autonomic nervous system.
(From Cannon, Mednick & Parnas, 1990b.)

There is a group of studies that have noted autonomic hyperresponsiveness
among high-risk children (Mednick & Schulsinger, 1968; Prentky, Salzman
& Klein, 1981; Van Dyke, Rosenthal & Rasmussen, 1974; Zahn, 1977).
Studies of schizophrenics have noted an autonomically hyperresponsive
subgroup among adult schizophrenics (Bartfai et al., 1987; Bartfai et al.,
1983; Frith et al., 1979). These autonomically hyperresponsive schizophrenics tend to evidence predominantly positive symptoms.

Among the hyperresponsive high-risk children there was a subgroup that
had suffered the most extremely stressful early rearing conditions of all the
high-risk children. Those high-risk subjects with stressful early rearing
conditions and with autonomic hyperresponsiveness evidenced significantly
elevated rates of predominantly positive-symptom schizophrenia (Cannon,
Mednick & Parnas, 1990b). It seems likely that the autonomic
hyperresponsiveness made these individuals vulnerable to these highly
stressful early experiences.

The base rate of predominantly positive-symptom schizophrenia in the
high-risk sample is 5%. Those with autonomic nervous system hyperresponsiveness and stressful early rearing conditions evidence a 40% rate of
positive-symptom schizophrenia (see Fig. 1.2).

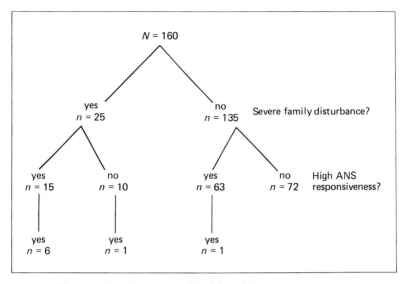

Figure 1.2 Decision-tree model of the etiology of predominantly positive-symptom schizophrenia in the high-risk group. ANS indicates autonomic nervous system. (From Cannon, Mednick & Parnas, 1990b.)

Conclusion

This introductory part of this volume is meant to illustrate the possible ways in which pre- and perinatal events may play a role in the etiology of adult schizophrenia. The remainder of the volume is divided into five parts. In Part II Nowakowski & Jones discuss basic knowledge concerning the development of the human and primate fetal brain. In Part III Nowakowski and Stagaard, Moos & Møllgård describe examples of genetic disturbances in brain development and possible genetic origins of a vulnerability to teratogenic agents. In Part IV, Mednick, Cannon & Barr review the literature on pre- and perinatal complications that are elevated in schizophrenics. Lyon & Barr consider areas of the brain which are at risk for pre- and perinatal damage. In part V Bogerts; Cannon; Breslin & Weinberger; Nasrallah, Schwarzkopf, Coffman & Olson provide a careful and complete review of neuropathology and structural brain imaging research on schizophrenics. It is interesting to compare these chapters with the Lyon & Barr chapter which enumerates the brain areas at particular risk of developmental damage and the two papers in Part II which describe the timetable and basic processes of brain development. Part VI attempts to integrate the basic fetal developmental research with the clinical and neuropathological and structural imaging research on schizophrenics.

This attempt to explain the complex syndromes of adult schizophrenia in terms of fetal developmental anomalies is a relatively new tack for behavioral science. It may go the way of earlier fads in psychiatric research. If that proves to be the case it is our hope that by focussing attention on errors in fetal neural development we will contribute to fostering basic knowledge on how the human brain grows and how that growth can be best protected.

At the moment, however, we judge that this enterprise merits intensified investigation in relation to schizophrenia. We cannot rule out the possibility that in the course of these studies we may discover that other behavioral deviations may have their roots in errors in the development of the fetal brain.

References

Barr, C. E., Mednick, S. A. & Munk-Jorgensen, P. (1990). Exposure to influenza epidemics during gestation and adult schizophrenia: A 40 year study. *Archives of General Psychiatry*, **47**, 869–74.

Bartfai, A., Levander, S., Edman, G., Schalling, D. & Sedvall, G. (1983). Skin conductance orienting responses in unmedicated recently admitted schizophrenic patients. *Psychophysiology*, **20**, 180–7.

Bartfai, A., Levander, S. E., Nyback, H. & Schalling, D. (1987). Skin conductance nonresponding and nonhabituation in schizophrenic patients. *Acta Psychiatrica Scandinavica*, **75**, 321–9.

Bogerts, B., Meertz, E. & Schonfeldt-Bausch, R. (1985). Basal ganglia and limbic system pathology in schizophrenia: A morphometric study of brain volume and shrinkage. *Archives of General Psychiatry*, **42**, 784–91.

Cannon, T. D., Fuhrmann, M., Mednick, S. A., Machon, R. A., Parnas, J. & Schulsinger, F. (1988). Third ventricle enlargement and reduced electrodermal responsiveness. *Psychophysiology*, **25**, 153–6.

Cannon, T. D., Mednick, S. & Parnas, J. (1989). Genetic and perinatal determinants of structural brain deficits in schizophrenia. *Archives of General Psychiatry*, **46**, 883–9.

Cannon, T. D., Mednick, S. A. & Parnas, J. (1990a). Two pathways to schizophrenia in children at risk. In L. Robins & M. Rutter (Eds.), *Straight and devious pathways from childhood to adulthood.* (pp. 328–50). Cambridge: Cambridge University Press.

Cannon, T. D., Mednick, S. A. & Parnas, J. (1990b). Antecedents of predominantly negative and predominantly positive symptom schizophrenia in a high-risk population. *Archives of General Psychiatry*, **47**, 622–32.

Darrow, C. W. (1937). Neural mechanisms controlling the palmar galvanic skin reflex and palmar sweating. *Archives of Neurological Psychiatry*, **37**, 641–63.

Frith, C. D., Stevens, M., Johnstone, E. C. & Crow, T. J. (1979). Skin conductance responsivity during acute episodes of schizophrenia as a predictor of symptomatic improvement. *Psychological Medicine*, **9**, 101–6.

Gottesman, I. I. & Shields, J. (1982). *Schizophrenia: The epigenetic puzzle.* Cambridge: Cambridge University Press.

Jakob, H. & Beckmann, H. (1986). Prenatal-developmental disturbances in the limbic allocortex in schizophrenia. *Biological Psychiatry*, **21**, 1181–3.

Kovelman, J. A. & Scheibel, A. B. (1984). A neurohistological correlate of schizophrenia. *Biological Psychiatry*, **19**, 1601–21.

Larsen, P. B., Schneiderman, N. & Pasin, R. D. (1986). Physiological bases of cardiovascular psychophysiology. In M. G. H. Coles, E. Doncin & S. W. Porges (Eds.), *Psychophysiology: Systems, processes, and applications.* New York: Guildford Press.

Machon, R. A., Mednick, S. A. & Huttunen, M. O. (1990). An update on the Helsinki influenza project. *Archives of General Psychiatry*, **47**, 292.

McNeil, T. F. (1988). Obstetric factors and perinatal injuries. In M. T. Tsuang & J. C. Simpson (Eds.), *Handbook of schizophrenia.* (pp. 319–44). Amsterdam: Elsevier.

Mednick, S. A., Machon, R. A., Huttunen, M. O. & Bonett, D. (1988). Adult schizophrenia following prenatal exposure to an influenza epidemic. *Archives of General Psychiatry*, **45**, 189–92.

Mednick, S. A. & Schulsinger, F. (1968). Some premorbid characteristics related to breakdown in children with schizophrenic mothers. *Journal of Psychiatric Research*, **6**, 267–91.

Parnas, J. (1985). Mates of schizophrenic mothers: A study of assortative mating from the American–Danish High Risk Study. *British Journal of Psychiatry*, **146**, 490–7.

Parnas, J., Schulsinger, F., Teasdale, T. W., Schulsinger, H., Feldman, P. M. & Mednick, S. A. (1982). Perinatal complications and clinical outcome within the schizophrenia spectrum. *British Journal of Psychiatry*, **140**, 416–20.

Prentky, R. A., Salzman, L. F. & Klein, R. H. (1981). Habituation and conditioning of skin conductance responses in children at risk. *Schizophrenia Bulletin*, **7**, 281–91.

Silverton, L., Finello, K. M., Mednick, S. A. & Schulsinger, F. (1985). Low birth weight and ventricular enlargement in a high-risk sample. *Journal of Abnormal Psychology*, **94**, 405–9.

Van Dyke, J. L., Rosenthal, D. & Rasmussen, P. V. (1974). Electrodermal functioning in adopted-away offspring of schizophrenics. *Journal of Psychiatric Research*, **10**, 199–215.

Venables, P. H. & Christie, M. J. (1973). Mechanisms instrumentation, recording techniques, and quantification of responses. In W. F. Prokasy & D. C. Raskin (Eds.), *Electrodermal activity in psychological research.* (pp. 2–124). New York: Academic Press.

Wang, G. H. (1964). *Neural control of sweating.* Madison, Wisconsin: University of Wisconsin Press.

Zahn, T. P. (1977). Autonomic nervous system characteristics possibly related to a genetic predisposition to schizophrenia. *Schizophrenia Bulletin*, **3**, 49–60.

13

Part II

Basic processes in fetal neural development

2

Some basic concepts of the development of the central nervous system

RICHARD S. NOWAKOWSKI

Robert Wood Johnson Medical School

Development of the neural tube

The development of the central nervous system (CNS) is a complicated, multi-step process. Early during the development of a vertebrate embryo, the CNS is formed from the primitive ectoderm by a process known as neurulation (Fig. 2.1), the result of which is the neural tube (Fig. 2.2). The lumen of the neural tube eventually becomes the ventricular system of the mature brain. The wall of the tube produces and becomes the cells and tissue of the mature brain.

Dimensional differentiation

The neural tube can be considered to have three dimensions – longitudinal, circumferential, and radial (Fig. 2.2). Differential differentiation along each of these dimensions during development is, to a substantial degree, responsible for the diverse anatomy of the mature brain. Differential differentiation along the longitudinal dimension produces the major subdivisions of the CNS (Fig. 2.3A). Within each of these major subdivisions, differential differentiation in the circumferential dimension gives rise to the development of structurally and functionally distinct areas. For example, in the spinal cord there are four circumferentially defined zones or plates: the roof plate, paired lateral plates, and the floor plate (Fig. 2.4). The lateral plate is usually divided by the sulcus limitans into a dorsally-positioned alar plate and a ventrally-positioned basal plate. The adult spinal cord is derived, for the most part,

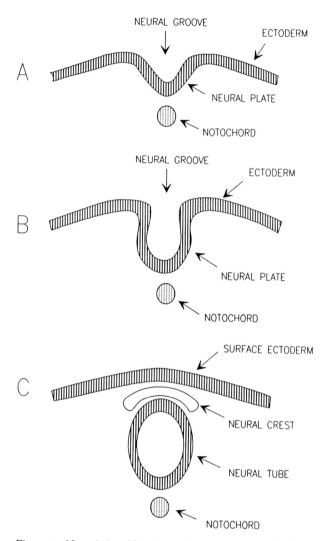

Figure 2.1 Neurulation. Neurulation begins near the end of the third week after conception. The ectoderm, which is the outer surface of the embryo, is induced to fold in upon itself to form the neural tube. A. At the beginning of neurulation there is a shallow groove just above the notochord; this shallow groove marks the position of the neural plate. B. As the neural groove deepens, the lateral edges of the neural plate fuse (C) to become the neural tube. The cells just lateral to the edge of the neural plate and some of the cells from the dorsal portion of the neural tube become the neural crest. The CNS is derived from the neural tube. The neural crest cells produce a variety of structures in the periphery, including most of the peripheral nervous system (LeDouarin, 1982).

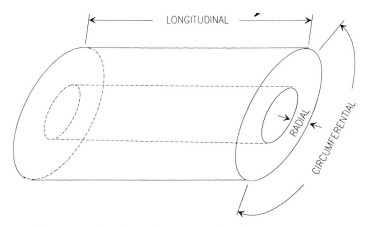

Figure 2.2. A caricature of the neural tube. The neural tube
has three dimensions: longitudinal, circumferential, and radial.
Differentiation along each of these three dimensions proceeds in
a different way. (See the text for further details.)

from the alar and basal plates, which become the dorsal and ventral horns of
the spinal cord, respectively. In more rostral portions of the nervous system,
the same four circumferential subdivisions exist; however, differential
development in the circumferential dimension produces a significantly
different adult morphology in each subdivision of the CNS. For example, in
the medulla the roof plate becomes wide, which displaces the alar and basal
plates laterally. Thus, in the adult, sensory and motor system derivatives of
the alar and basal plates are also pushed aside as a consequence of the
expansion of the roof plate and are oriented mediolaterally around the sulcus
limitans rather than dorsoventrally as in the spinal cord. The significance of
this circumferential differentiation is that it *precedes* the functional organization of the nervous system into sensory and motor subdivisions. In other
parts of the nervous system, such anatomical differentiation also seems to
precede functional differentiation. One example is the developing hippocampal region, in which future cytoarchitectonic subdivisions can be
detected before the first neurons to comprise them have been generated
(Nowakowski & Rakic, 1979).

It should be emphasized that differentiation in both the longitudinal and
circumferential dimensions suggests that different portions of the wall of the
neural tube, even at early stages, have different potential and developmental
capabilities (Rakic & Goldman-Rakic, 1982; Rakic, 1988). Thus, the basic
organizational plan of the nervous system is defined early during development by differentiation along the length and circumference of the neural
tube.

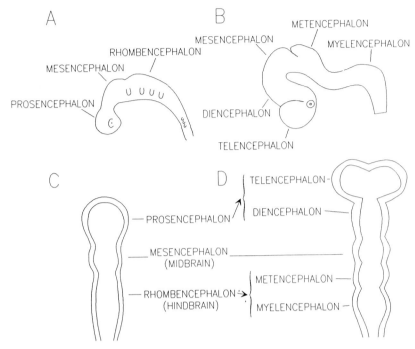

Figure 2.3. Longitudinal differentiation of the neural tube.
Differential differentiation along the longitudinal axis produces
the major subdivisions of the CNS. In a four-week-old human
embryo there are three primary brain vesicles: the
prosencephalon, mesencephalon, and rhombencephalon (A, C).
In the next week or two the primary vesicles become
subdivided. The prosencephalon becomes the telencephalon
and diencephalon, and the rhombencephalon becomes the
metencephalon and myelencephalon (B, D).

Neuronal proliferation, migration, and differentiation

Additional structural refinement and differentiation in the internal organization of each CNS subdivision is, for the most part, the result of a series of
changes in the radial dimension which produce a variety of laminar schemes
in different parts of the neural tube. To understand the variety of laminar
organizational schemes which exist in the different parts of the adult CNS, it
is necessary to understand three distinctly different cellular processes: cell
proliferation, cell migration, and cell differentiation. Together, these three
steps can be considered to comprise the 'life history' of a single neuron or glial

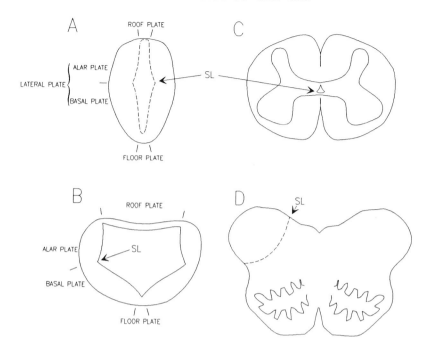

Figure 2.4. Circumferential differentiation of the neural tube. In the spinal cord there are four circumferential zones or plates: a floor plate; an alar plate; a basal plate; and a roof plate. The names of these plates are derived from their position around the tube; (the Latin word *ala*, means wing). In the medulla, the alar and basal plates are displaced laterally by the widening and attenuation of the roof plate. In both the spinal cord and medulla the sulcus limitans marks the border between the basal and alar plates, and in the adult the morphological relationship between the sensory and motor derivatives of the alar and basal plates is similar, although their orientation around the sulcus limitans shifts from dorsoventral in the spinal cord to mediolateral in the medulla.

cell; each cell must pass successively through all three of these steps in order to become a mature component of the CNS. Cell proliferation, cell migration, and cell differentiation occur simultaneously within every division and subdivision of the developing CNS, but for a single cell these steps represent a cascade of developmental events. Cells which pass through the cascade early can influence the fate of those cells which subsequently pass through the cascade. In other words, through intercellular interactions cells present in the same part of the nervous system, in the same or even in different states of maturation, can interact and affect each other's fate.

Cell proliferation

It appears that all of the neurons of primate, including human, CNS are produced during the developmental period, which probably extends to only about 3–6 months after birth; there have, however, been reports of neuron production in the adult canary (Goldman & Nottebohm, 1983; Nottebohm, 1985) and also in the adult rat (Bayer, 1982; Bayer, Yackel & Puri, 1982; Kaplan, 1977; Kaplan & Hinds, 1977). For the most part there is no proliferation of neurons in the adult primate CNS (Nowakowski & Rakic, 1981; Rakic, 1982, 1985, 1988). In the developing CNS cell proliferation occurs, for the most part, in two specialized zones which line the ventricular system (Fig. 2.5). The first of these two zones to appear is the ventricular zone (Boulder Committee, 1970), which is a pseudostratified columnar epithelium. All parts of the developing CNS have a ventricular zone and, in some parts, the ventricular zone is the *only* proliferative zone to appear. In other parts of the developing CNS a second proliferative zone appears. This zone, known as the subventricular zone, differs in a number of ways from the ventricular zone. For example, the cells of the ventricular zone and subventricular zone differ from one another in their mode of proliferation (see legend for Fig. 2.5 for details). It has been speculated (see Nowakowski, 1987; Nowakowski & Rakic, 1981) that the subventricular zone is a phylogenetically 'newer' feature. For example, all of the neurons of the major subdivisions (areas CA1, CA2, and CA3) of the hippocampus, which is classified as an archicortical or 'old' cortical structure, are derived from the ventricular zone (Nowakowski & Rakic, 1981). In contrast, a substantial subventricular zone is present in the developing neocortex, and is believed to contribute large numbers of neurons to that phylogenetically newer cortex, (Nowakowski & Rakic, 1981). A similar developmental scheme seems to exist in the developing diencephalon (Rakic, 1977). Again, these differences in the distribution of the two proliferative zones along the ventricular surface appear early, just as the first neurons are being produced (Nowakowski & Rakic, 1981); this indicates that the ventricular surface of the developing nervous system is a mosaic, and that the development of major subdivisions of the CNS follows distinctly different patterns even at early stages.

Cell migration

While cell proliferation occurs in areas adjacent to the ventricular surface, in many portions of the adult nervous system neurons are located at quite a distance from the ventricular surface. Therefore, a mechanism for the movement of cells from their site of proliferation to their ultimate position is necessary. There are two basic but very different ways that neurons make this movement. The first does not seem to require active locomotory movement by the post-mitotic neuron. In this case a postmitotic neuron leaves the proliferative population (influenced to do so by some unknown signal or signals) and is displaced only a very short distance from the border of the proliferative zone. Shortly thereafter, as the next post-mitotic neurons are similarly displaced outward from the proliferative zone, the original cells are displaced slightly further. This type of cell movement is generally considered to be passive cell displacement (Fig. 2.6). The second way that young neurons move from the proliferative zone to their ultimate positions requires the active participation of the postmitotic neurons in producing their own displacement. In this case, neurons leave the proliferative zone and move a great distance through the intermediate zone, with progressively later-generated neurons in many instances bypassing neurons produced earlier (Fig. 2.7). This active process of cell movement is generally referred to as neuronal migration (for review see Sidman & Rakic, 1973) and takes place in the cerebral cortex (both archicortex and neocortex).

Outside-to-inside spatiotemporal gradient. In those parts of the CNS in which passive cell displacement occurs, neurons that leave the proliferative population earliest are, in general, those that are ultimately located furthest from the proliferative zone. The subsequently-generated neurons are found at levels progressively closer to the proliferative zone (Fig. 2.6). Thus, there is a correlation between the final position of a neuron and its time of origin. For areas in which there is passive cell displacement, this correlation is referred to as an 'outside-to-inside' spatiotemporal gradient. Outside and inside are both defined with respect to the position of the cells relative to the proliferative zone; for the most part, outside refers to the pial surface, and inside refers to the ventricular surface. Areas of the nervous system in which the outside-to-inside spatiotemporal gradient is manifest include the thalamus (Altman & Bayer, 1979; Angevine, 1970; Rakic, 1977), the hypothalamus (Ifft, 1972), spinal cord (Nornes & Das, 1974), many regions of the brainstem (Altman & Bayer, 1981; Taber-Pierce, 1972), the retina (Sidman, 1961; Walsh *et al.*, 1983), and the dentate gyrus of the hippocampal formation (Angevine, 1965; Bayer, 1982; Bayer *et al.*, 1982; Nowakowski & Rakic, 1981; Wyss & Sripanidkulchai, 1985).

Inside-to-outside spatiotemporal gradient. In those parts of the developing CNS in which the migrating young neurons actively contribute to their own displacement away from the proliferative zones, the result is an 'inside-to-outside' spatiotemporal gradient. In this pattern, the earliest-generated cells

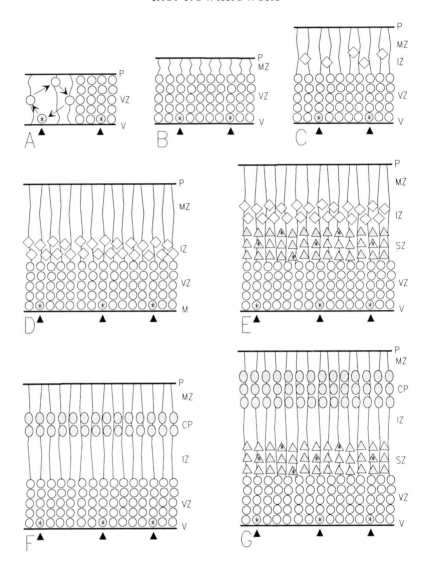

Figure 2.5. Differentiation in the radial dimension. In A, B and C the early stages of the differentiation of the neural tube are shown. All parts of the early developing CNS have a ventricular zone (VZ) and eventually develop a marginal zone (MZ) just subjacent to the pial surface (P). In the ventricular zone the nuclei of the cells are stratified, but each cell has contacts that reach the ventricular (V) and pial surfaces (P) of the neural tube. The left side of drawing A illustrates the movement of a single cell as it passes through the various phases of the cell cycle; DNA synthesis occurs in the outer half of the ventricular zone and mitosis (i.e. cell division) occurs adjacent to the ventricular surface. This movement of the cell's nucleus is known as interkinetic nuclear migration. Shortly after neurulation the neural tube consists of only the ventricular zone. The next zone to appear (B) is the marginal zone, which is an almost cell-free zone just subjacent to the pial surface. Shortly after the formation of the marginal zone an intermediate zone (IZ) forms; this zone contains the first post-mitotic cells of the nervous system. The IZ is located between the VZ and MZ. D, E, F and G illustrate various alternatives for the subsequent radial development of the CNS. D: In some parts of the neural tube the only proliferative zone present is the ventricular zone. The post-mitotic cells derived from the VZ aggregate and mature in the IZ, just adjacent to the VZ. One portion of the nervous system which has this pattern of radial differentiation is the spinal cord. E: In other portions of the nervous system post-mitotic cells also aggregate in the IZ and differentiate there, but some of these cells are derived from the subventricular zone (SZ). The dorsal thalamus is an example of a portion of the nervous system that follows this pattern of development. F and G: Examples of cortical regions. In the hippocampus (F) all of the post-mitotic cells are derived from the VZ. They migrate across the sparsely populated IZ and form a cortical plate (CP). In the neocortex (G) both a VZ and a SZ are present. Again the derivatives of these two proliferative zones migrate across the IZ and form a cortical plate. Abbreviations: V, ventricular surface; VZ, ventricular zone; SZ, subventricular zone; IZ, intermediate zone; CP, cortical plate; MZ, marginal zone; P, pial surface.

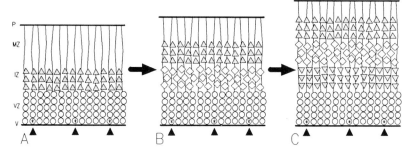

Figure 2.6. In some areas of the developing nervous system cell movement is by passive displacement. Some cells leave the proliferative zone and take up a position only a short distance from the proliferative zone. Later, as other cells are produced by the proliferative zone, the earlier produced cells are displaced outward. Diagrams A through C illustrate the progressive passive displacement of previously generated neurons away from the ventricular surface by subsequently later generated neurons. A: The earliest generated neurons to leave the ventricular zone are shown as triangles. B: The next group of neurons to be generated are represented by diamonds. Their movement out of the ventricular zone displaces the earlier generated neurons towards the pial surface. C: The last neurons generated, represented by inverted triangles, displace both of the earlier generated populations of neurons. This sequence of events produces a specific distribution of neurons known as an outside-to-inside spatiotemporal gradient. Abbreviations: V, ventricular surface; VZ, ventrical zone; IZ, intermediate zone; MZ, marginal zone; P, pial surface.

remain closest to the proliferative zone and comprise the deepest layers while the latest-generated cells move farthest from the proliferative zone and occupy the most superficial layers. Inside-to-outside spatiotemporal gradients are found in most portions of the cerebral cortex (Angevine, 1965; Angevine & Sidman, 1961; Caviness, 1982; Caviness & Sidman, 1973; Hinds, 1968; Miller, 1985, 1987; Rakic, 1975b; Rakic & Nowakowski, 1981; Wyss & Sripanidkulchai, 1985) and in several subcortical areas (Cooper & Rakic, 1981; Hickey & Hitchcock, 1968). Areas in which spatiotemporal gradients of the inside-to-outside type occur are, in general, well-laminated structures in that they have tangentially oriented layers that run parallel with the surface of the proliferative zones. During their migration many neurons are guided to their final position by radial glial fibers (Rakic, 1971, 1972), which provide the scaffolding for the future adult neocortex and for other cortical and non-cortical structures as well (Nowakowski & Rakic, 1979; Rakic, 1971, 1978, 1982; Rakic et al., 1974; Eckenhoff & Rakic, 1984). It has also been speculated that radial fibers provide the scaffolding for the columnar organization of the

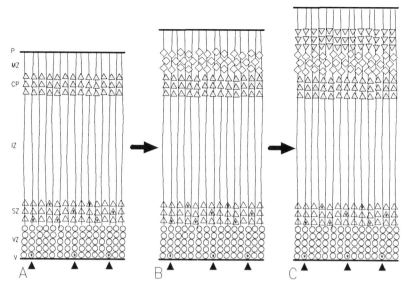

Figure 2.7. The sequence of events associated with active neuronal migration. In some parts of the developing CNS, neurons leaving the proliferative zone move a great distance before taking up their final position. The sequence of events involved in this process is illustrated in A, B and C. A: The first neurons to leave the proliferative zone (triangles) assemble in a formation known as a cortical plate, which is situated between the intermediate and marginal zones. B: The next group of neurons to be generated (diamonds) leaves the proliferative population and moves across the intermediate zone and past the earlier generated cells to take up a position on the top of the cortical plate. C: The last generated neurons (inverted triangles) migrate across the intermediate zone and past both groups of earlier generated cells to take up residence at the top of the cortical plate. This type of distribution of neurons is known as an inside-to-outside spatiotemporal gradient. Abbreviations: V, ventricular surface; VZ, ventricular zone; SZ, subventricular zone; IZ, intermediate zone; CP, cortical plate; MZ, marginal zone; P, pial surface.

adult cortex (Eckenhoff & Rakic, 1984; Mountcastle, 1978; Rakic, 1978, 1982, 1988; Smart & McSherry, 1982). The process of neuronal migration (Fig. 2.8) is a complicated one and consists of at least three phases (for review see Nowakowski, 1985). The three phases are: initiation of migration; a locomotory phase; and a termination phase. In the initiation phase a young neuron starts its migration by leaving the proliferative population; during this phase, a cell in the proliferating population makes the transition from neuroblast (i.e. a proliferating cell) to young neuron (i.e. a non-proliferating,

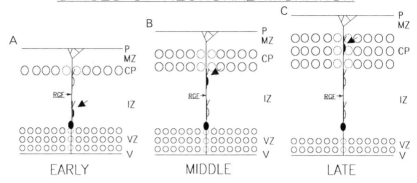

Figure 2.8. A schematic illustration of the interaction between migrating neurons and radial glial fibers. After leaving the proliferative zone, the young neuron is guided by a radially aligned glial cell as it moves towards its final position in the cortical plate. The progression of one such young neuron from the proliferative zone through the intermediate zone to the cortical plate is illustrated by a single black cell arrowed in each of the three drawings A, B and C. The migratory process can be divided into three stages. First (A), as a young neuron leaves the proliferative population it becomes apposed to a radial glial fiber and acquires a polarity directed toward the pial surface (P). Next (B), it enters the locomotory phase and traverses the intermediate zone (IZ), maintaining its apposition to the radial glial fiber and its polarity as it moves through the zone. Later (C), when it reaches the top of the cortical plate (CP), it loses its apposition to the radial glial fiber and reorganizes its polarity in order to differentiate into a mature neuron. Disruption of any of the three steps of the migratory process can result in ectopic neurons. Other abbreviations: V, ventricular surface; VZ, ventricular zone; CP, cortical plate; MZ, marginal zone; RGF, radial glial fibre.

permanently postmitotic cell). The young neuron becomes apposed to a radial glial fiber and establishes an axis of polarity away from the ventricular surface. Once aligned with the radial glial fiber the second, or locomotory, phase of migration begins. During this phase, a young neuron moves actively along the surface of a radial glial cell, retaining its apposition to the radial glial fiber and its axis of polarity directed away from the proliferative zone. In the cerebral cortex the locomotory phase can be very long, and a migrating neuron can move along a radial glial fiber which may be tens of millimeters long. Once it reaches the vicinity of its final position, a migrating young neuron must stop its migration and become detached from the radial glial fiber. At this point the young neuron can continue its differentiation process by growing dendrites and sending out axons that eventually make contacts with other neurons.

Disruptions of cell position. If any of the three phases which comprise the process of neuronal migration is disrupted, an *abnormality in cell position results*. Neurons that fail to reach their appropriate position are said to be ectopic (or heterotopic) (Rakic, 1975a). Neuropathologists have described a variety of defects in cell position. In humans, the best studied examples of defects in neuronal positioning are in the cerebral cortex, where abnormalities in neuronal migration have been associated with a variety of diseases and syndromes ranging from extremely severe mental retardation and failure to thrive to 'rather minor' behavioral disorders. Some of the behavioral disorders that have been associated with the disruption of the migratory process include schizophrenia and dyslexia. In the case of schizophrenia, Kovelman and Scheibel (1984, 1986) have presented evidence for the existence of ectopic neurons in area CA1 of the hippocampus of brains of patients with severe schizophrenia. In the case of dyslexia, Galaburda, Sherman, and Geschwind (1983) have demonstrated islands of ectopic neurons in the brains of several humans with severe dyslexia. In addition, a number of more severe disorders associated with disruptions of the migratory process include hydrocephalus, methanol exposure, mental retardation, seizures, lissencephaly, methylmercury poisoning, and craniofacial anomalies (Choi & Kudo, 1981; Evrard *et al.*, 1978; Mikhael & Mattar, 1978; Miller, 1986; Richman *et al.*, 1975; Zimmerman, Bilaniuk & Grossman, 1983).

From human pathological data it is difficult to learn the developmental fate of neurons that fail to migrate to their proper positions. It is not known, for example, if these abnormally-positioned neurons make connections with the rest of the brain; nor is it known whether any connections they do make are with their normal targets or some other targets. Most importantly it is not known how these abnormalities in connectivity (if they exist) might affect the function of the area of the brain in which these cells were normally destined to reside. Some insight into these issues is coming from studies in mutant mice that have defects in neuronal migration (presented elsewhere in this volume, Nowakowski, 1990).

Cell differentiation

The final phase in the life history of a neuron is its differentiation. This is an extraordinarily complex process that is responsible for a large proportion of the diversity, in all its many aspects, of the adult CNS. During the differentiation of a neuron, axonal and dendritic processes are elaborated, and neurotransmitter phenotypes are expressed. In many cases, the axon grows a long distance over a complicated terrain until it reaches its final target. The dendrites grow out and form a characteristic arborization pattern for each particular cell class. The specific neurotransmitter enzymes that are characteristic of that cell class are also produced; in addition to elaborating the specific enzymes to produce neurotransmitters, neurons must also produce at each postsynaptic site the specific receptors it needs to receive input from its various presynaptic partners. Also, some neurons will elaborate a signal which causes their axon to become myelinated; others will not. As neurons acquire their mature properties, glial cells also differentiate into various forms; some become oligodendrocytes that produce myelin, others become astrocytes that perform other functions (Temple & Raff, 1986; ffrench-Constant & Raff, 1986). In humans, it is known that the myelination of most pathways in the CNS continues long after birth (for review see Richardson, 1982). In fact Flechsig (1920), in his classical work on myelination in the developing human cerebral cortex, established the basis of the traditional classification of neocortical areas into primary, secondary and association cortices. The complexity of the process of cell differentiation in the CNS, as outlined briefly above, is beyond the scope of this review; therefore, the discussion below will be confined to the limited aspect of axon–target interactions. For other topics the reader is referred to recent reviews (Easter et al., 1985; Jacobson, 1978; Jonakait & Black, 1986; Purves & Lichtman, 1985; Wiesel, 1982).

Axon–target interactions. As an axon in the CNS grows, it extends its process from the cell soma to a target or postsynaptic cell. In so doing, the axon must find its way through a complicated terrain to the area of its potential target. Once there it must not only select the appropriate target cell but also find the appropriate part of the dendritic tree of the appropriate target cell in order to make its synapses. Clearly a variety of mechanisms are required in order to make this complicated process successful. Recently, it has become evident that many axons in the developing CNS do not grow directly to their final targets but instead grow 'exuberantly'. Thus, axons can transiently innervate both areas of the nervous system and specific cells that they do not normally contact in the adult. Two types of transient connections are made: divergent and convergent (see Fig. 2.9). Divergence means that, during development, one axon or one neuron innervates a greater area or number of cells than it normally does in the adult (Fig. 2.9A). At a later stage of development the extra collaterals of the divergently-projecting population of axons are eliminated, thereby reducing the projection area to its normal adult size (Fig. 2.9A'). Convergence is the converse of divergence. This

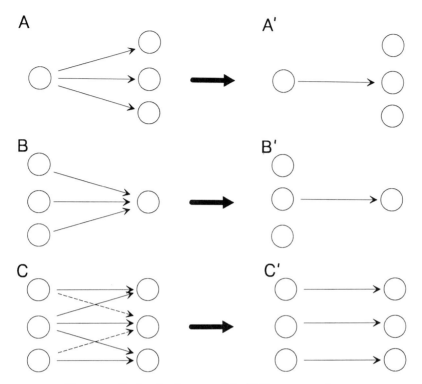

Figure 2.9. During development of the CNS two types of exuberant connections occur. A. Transient *divergence*: A single source of axons (either a single cell or a single population of neurons) projects to an area broader than its eventual adult distribution. A subsequent withdrawal of a portion of the projection produces the adult pattern (A'). B. Transient *convergence*: Axonal projections from more than one source (i.e. from more than one cell or population of neurons) terminate on a single target. Subsequent withdrawal of the projection from some of the sources produces the adult pattern (B'). C. Transient *divergence* and *convergence* in combination: In this situation some exuberant projections of both types must be withdrawn to produce the adult pattern of connections (C').

means that during development one target neuron can be innervated by several axons (Fig. 2.9B), even though in the adult only one of these axons might innervate that target (Fig. 2.9B'). Divergent and convergent transient axonal projections are not mutually exclusive, and it is probable that both occur within single populations of neurons (Fig. 2.9C). If and when this is the case, both extra divergent and convergent axonal projections would have to be eliminated in order to establish the adult pattern of connections (Fig. 2.9C').

Axon elimination. The mechanism by which the extra axonal connections are eliminated is unclear. Two distinctly different regressive phenomena appear to be responsible: naturally-occurring neuronal death, and the reorganization of axonal and dendritic trees (Cowan *et al.*, 1984; Innocenti, Clarke & Kraftsik, 1986; Segraves & Innocenti, 1985). Divergent connections seem to be able to be eliminated via two mechanisms. First, in the case of a *single* neuron projecting to a wider target than it does in the adult, the removal of the transient connection seems to occur either by retraction of the neuron's axon collaterals or, perhaps, by a shrinking of the terminal arbor of the axon. Second, in the case of a *population* of neurons projecting to a wider target than in the adult, the transient connections can be removed by a process of selective cell death, in which those neurons which project beyond the normal adult innervation territory die. Examples of the occurrence of both of these mechanisms are known. It is known for example, that during the development of the visual cortex, pyramidal neurons in the visual cortex send transient collaterals to the spinal cord, which they do not normally innervate in the adult animal. Later in development, this transient innervation is eliminated by retraction of the spinal collaterals of these axons while their cells of origin persist (O'Leary & Stanfield, 1985; Stanfield & O'Leary, 1985a, 1985b). The occurrence of extensive neuronal cell death during development has also been well documented, and it has been hypothesized (Cowan *et al.*, 1984; Oppenheim, 1981) that naturally-occurring neuronal death contributing to the elimination of divergently-projecting collaterals is a mechanism of error correction. It has also been suggested that convergent projections can be eliminated by means of naturally-occurring cell death (Cowan *et al.*, 1984; Oppenheim, 1981). In addition, elimination of extra convergent projections seems to involve a retraction of the terminal synaptic field of surviving neurons (Cowan *et al.*, 1984; Oppenheim, 1981; Wiesel, 1982). Thus, although development of a complex organ such as the nervous system is generally considered to be a series of *progressive events*, axonal elimination and neuronal cell death are major *regressive events* which occur normally during the development of the CNS (Heffner, Lumsden & O'Leary, 1990; O'Leary, 1987; Purves *et al.*, 1987; Purves, Snider & Voyvodic, 1988).

Biological control of these regressive events is generally believed to involve a number of factors alone or in combination; these include competition either for limited synaptic space or for usage of growth factors and the interaction of different neurons by means of electrical activity (Fawcett, O'Leary & Cowan, 1984; Henderson *et al.*, 1986; Purves & Lichtman, 1985; Schmidt, 1985a, 1985b; Schmidt & Tieman, 1985; Toulouse, Dehane & Changeux, 1986). It seems likely that all of these mechanisms will be found to contribute to the

32

elimination of transient exuberant connections (e.g. Easter *et al.*, 1985). In addition to the loss of axons and axon collaterals (Crespo, O'Leary & Cowan, 1985; Rakic & Riley, 1983), the elimination of transient connections also involves a net decrease in numbers of synapses and synaptic densities (Oppenheim, 1981; Rakic *et al.*, 1986). One suggestion (Rakic *et al.*, 1986) is that the emergence of a full complement of functional behavioural repertoire involves not only the elimination of excess synapses but also the acquisition of synaptic efficiency at the molecular level and the reorganization of synapses without a concomitant increase in their numbers. A variety of processes are likely to be involved in controlling this aspect of the differentiation of the nervous system, including steroidal hormones (Arnold & Breedlove, 1985; Arnold & Gorski, 1984; Nordeen *et al.*, 1985), and the remodeling of such processes may continue on into adulthood (Nottebohm, 1985; Purves & Hadley, 1985; Toulouse *et al.*, 1986). The existence of regressive processes such as neuronal death, the retraction of exuberant collaterals, and the elimination of synapses during CNS development is likely to play a role in a variety of human disorders, including dyslexia (Galaburda *et al.*, 1983; Kemper, 1984), schizophrenia (Kovelman & Scheibel, 1984, 1986), fetal alcohol syndrome (Miller, 1986, 1987), methylmercury poisoning (Choi *et al.*, 1978) and others (e.g. Choi & Kudo, 1981; Otake & Schull, 1984; Zimmerman *et al.*, 1983). In each of these syndromes the process of neuronal migration seems to have been disrupted in some way. The presumption is that in these disorders normal functional competence is not achieved, at least in part because the abnormally-positioned neurons produced from the disruption of neuronal migration do not make normal connections. The exact relationship between the severity of the functional compromise and abnormal neuronal position is not clear at this time; however, it seems reasonable to speculate that those populations of ectopic neurons that during development are normally innervated by divergent, exuberantly projecting axon collaterals are more likely to become normally innervated by the axons which would have found them had they been in their normal position. Thus, such neurons are more likely to be able to participate in normal function. Testing this hypothesis in humans is obviously not possible, but there are a variety of ways of producing abnormally-positioned neurons in experimental animals by genetic means (e.g. Caviness & Rakic, 1978; Nowakowski, 1985, 1988; Nowakowski & Wahlsten, 1985a, 1985b; Pearlman, 1985) and by other experimental avenues (Miller, 1987) that may provide a useful way to test this speculation. An examination of these issues is given elsewhere in this volume (see Chapter 4).

References

Altman, J. & Bayer, S. A. (1979). Development of the diencephalon in the rat: V. Thymidine-radiographic observations on internuclear and intranuclear gradients in the thalamus. *Journal of Comparative Neurology*, **188**, 473–500.

Altman, J. & Bayer, S. A. (1981). Development of the brain stem in the rat: V. Thymidine-radiographic study of the time of origin of neurons in the midbrain tegmentum. *Journal of Comparative Neurology*, **198**, 677–716.

Angevine, J. B., Jr. (1965). Time of neuron origin in the hippocampal region: An autoradiographic study in the mouse. *Experimental Neurology (Supplement)*, **2**, 1–71.

(1970). Time of neuron origin in the diencephalon of the mouse: An autoradiographic study. *Journal of Comparative Neurology*, **139**, 129–88.

Angevine, J. B., Jr. & Sidman, R. L. (1961). Autoradiographic study of cell migration during histogenesis of cerebral cortex in the mouse. *Nature, London*, **192**, 766–8.

Arnold, A. P. & Breedlove, S. M. (1985). Organizational and activational effects of sex steroids on brain and behavior: A reanalysis. *Hormones and Behavior*, **19**, 469–98.

Arnold, A. P. & Gorski, R. A. (1984). Gonadal steroid induction of structural sex differences in the central nervous system. *Annual Review of Neuroscience*, **7**, 413–42.

Bayer, S. A. (1982). Changes in the total number of dentate granule cells in juvenile and adult rats: A correlated volumetric and ^{3}H-thymidine autoradiographic study. *Experimental Brain Research*, **46**, 315–23.

Bayer, S. A., Yackel, J. W. & Puri, P. S. (1982). Neurons in the rat dentate gyrus granular layer substantially increase during juvenile and adult life. *Science*, **216**, 890–2.

Boulder Committee (1970). Embryonic vertebrate central nervous system: Revised terminology. *Anatomical Record*, **166**, 257–61.

Caviness, V. S., Jr. (1982). Neocortical histogenesis in normal and reeler mice: A developmental study based on [^{3}H]thymidine autoradiography. *Developmental Brain Research*, **4**, 293–302.

Caviness, V. S., Jr. & Rakic, P. (1978). Mechanisms of cortical development: A view from mutations in mice. *Annual Review of Neuroscience*, **1**, 297–326.

Caviness, V. S., Jr. & Sidman, R. L. (1973). Time of origin of corresponding cell classes in the cerebral cortex of normal and reeler mutant mice: An autoradiographic analysis. *Journal of Comparative Neurology*, **148**, 141–52.

Choi, B. H. & Kudo, M. (1981). Abnormal migration and gliomatosis in epidermal nevus syndrome. *Acta Neuropathologica*, **53**, 319–25.

Choi, B. H., Lapham, L. W., Amin-Zaki, L. & Saleem, T. (1978). Abnormal neuronal migration, deranged cerebral cortical organization, and diffuse white matter astrocytosis of human fetal brain: A major effect of methylmercury poisoning *in utero*. *Journal of Neuropathology and Experimental Neurology*, **37**, 719–33.

Cooper, M. L. & Rakic, P. (1981). Neurogenetic gradients in the superior and inferior colliculi of the rhesus monkey. *Journal of Comparative Neurology*, **202**, 309–34.

Cowan, W. M., Fawcett, J. W., O'Leary, D. D. & Stanfield, B. B. (1984). Regressive events in neurogenesis. *Science*, **225**, 1258–65.

Crespo, D., O'Leary, D. D. & Cowan, W. M. (1985). Changes in the numbers of optic nerve fibers during late prenatal and postnatal development in the albino rat. *Brain Research*, **351**, 129–34.

Easter, S. S., Jr., Purves, D., Rakic, P. & Spitzer, N. C. (1985). The changing view of neural specificity. *Science*, **230**, 507–11.

Eckenhoff, M. F. & Rakic, P. (1984). Radial organization of the hippocampal dentate gyrus: A Golgi, ultrastructural and immunocytochemical analysis in the developing rhesus monkey. *Journal of Comparative Neurology*, **223**, 1–21.

Evrard, P., Caviness, V. S., Jr., Prats-Vinas, J. & Lyon, G. (1978). The mechanism of arrest of neuronal migration in the Zellweger malformation: An hypothesis based upon cytoarchitectonic analysis. *Acta Neuropathologica*, **41**, 109–17.

Fawcett, J. W., O'Leary, D. D. & Cowan, W. M. (1984). Activity and the control of ganglion cell death in the rat retina. *Proceedings of the National Academy of Sciences, USA*, **81**, 5589–93.

Flechsig, P. (1920). *Anatomie des menschlichen Gehirns und Ruckenmarks auf myelogenetischer Grundlage*. Leipzig: Georg Theime.

ffrench-Constant, C. & Raff, M. C. (1986). Proliferating bipotential glial progenitor cells in adult rat optic nerve. *Nature, London*, **319**, 499–502.

Galaburda, A. M., Sherman, G. F. & Geschwind, N. (1983). Developmental dyslexia: Third consecutive case with cortical anomalies. *Society for Neuroscience Abstracts*, **9**, 940.

Goldman, S. A. & Nottebohm, F. (1983). Neuronal production, migration, and differentiation in a vocal control nucleus of the adult female canary brain. *Proceedings of the National Academy of Sciences, USA*, **80**, 2390–4.

Heffner, C. D., Lumsden, A. G. & O'Leary, D. D. (1990). Target control of collateral extension 'and directional axon growth in the mammalian brain. *Science*, **247**, 217–20.

Henderson, C. E., Benoit, P., Huchet, M., Guenet, J. L. & Changeux, J. P. (1986). Increase of neurite-promoting activity for spinal neurons in muscles of 'paralyse' mice and tenotomised rats. *Brain Research*, **390**, 65–70.

Hickey, T. L. & Hitchcock, P. F. (1968). Neurogenesis in the cat lateral geniculate nucleus: A ^{3}H–thymidine study. *Journal of Comparative Neurology*, **228**, 186–99.

Hinds, J. W. (1968). Autoradiographic study of histogenesis in the mouse olfactory bulb: I. Time of origin of neurons and neuroglia. *Journal of Comparative Neurology*, **134**, 287–304.

Ifft, J. D. (1972). An autoradiographic study of the time of final division of neurons in the rat hypothalamic nuclei. *Journal of Comparative Neurology*, **144**, 193–204.

Innocenti, G. M., Clarke, S. & Kraftsik, R. (1986). Interchange of callosal and association projections in the developing visual cortex. *The Journal of Neuroscience*, **6**, 1384–409.

Jacobson, M. (1978). *Developmental Neurobiology*. New York: Plenum.

Jonakait, G. M. & Black, I. B. (1986). Neurotransmitter phenotypic plasticity in the mammalian embryo. *Current Topics in Developmental Biology*, **20**, 165–75.

Kaplan, M. S. (1977). Neurogenesis in the 3-month-old rat visual cortex. *Journal of Comparative Neurology*, **195**, 323–38.

Kaplan, M. S. & Hinds, J. W. (1977). Neurogenesis in the adult rat: Electron microscopic analysis of light radioautographs. *Science*, **197**, 1092–4.

Kemper, T. L. (1984). Asymmetrical lesions in dyslexia. In N. Geschwind & A. M. Galaburda (Eds), *Cerebral Dominance: The Biological Foundations* (pp. 75–89). Cambridge, Massachusetts: Harvard University Press.

Kovelman, J. A. & Scheibel, A. B. (1984). A neurohistological correlate of schizophrenia. *Biological Psychiatry*, **19**, 1601–21.

Kovelman, J. A. & Scheibel, A. B. (1986). Biological substrates of schizophrenia. *Acta Neurologica Scandinavica*, **73**, 1–32.

LeDouarin, N. (1982). *The Neural Crest*. Cambridge: Cambridge University Press.

Mikhael, M. A. & Mattar, A. G. (1978). Malformation of the cerebral cortex with heterotopia of the gray matter. *Journal of Computer Assisted Tomography*, **2**, 291–6.

Miller, M. W. (1985). Cogeneration of retrogradely labeled corticocortical projection and GABA-immunoreactive local circuit neurons in cerebral cortex. *Developmental Brain Research*, **23**, 187–92.

Miller, M. W. (1986). Effects of alcohol on the generation and migration of cerebral cortical neurons. *Science*, **233**, 1308–11.

Miller, M. W. (1987). The effect of prenatal exposure to alcohol on the distribution and the time of origin of corticospinal neurons in the rat. *Journal of Comparative Neurology*, **257**, 372–82.

Mountcastle, V. B. (1978). An organizing principle for cerebral function: The unit module and distributed system. In G. Edelman & V. B. Mountcastle (Eds), *The Mindful Brain* (pp. 7–50). Cambridge, Massachusetts: MIT Press.

Nordeen, E. J. Nordeen, K. W., Sengelaub, D. R. & Arnold, A. P. (1985). Androgens prevent normally occurring cell-death in a sexually dimorphic spinal nucleus. *Science*, **229**, 671–3.

Nornes, H. L. & Das, G. D. (1974). Temporal patterns of neurons in spinal cord of rat: I. An autoradiographic study – time and sites of origin and migration and settling pattern of neuroblasts. *Brain Research*, **73**, 121–38.

Nottebohm, F. (1985). Neuronal replacement in adulthood. *Annals of the New York Academy of Sciences*, **457**, 143–61.

Nowakowski, R. S. (1985). Neuronal migration in the hippocampal lamination defect (Hld) mutant mouse. In H. J. Marthy (Ed.), *Cellular and Molecular Control of Direct Cell Interactions* (pp. 133–54). New York: Plenum.

(1987). Basic Concepts of CNS development. *Child Development*, **58**, 568–95.

(1988). Development of the hippocampal formation in mutant mice. *Drug Development Research*, **15**, 315–36.

Nowakowski, R. S. & Rakic, P. (1979). The mode of migration of neurons to the hippocampus. A Golgi and electron microscopic analysis in foetal rhesus monkey. *Journal of Neurocytology*, **8**, 697–718.

(1981). The site of origin and route and rate of migration of neurons to the hippocampal region of the rhesus monkey. *Journal of Comparative Neurology*, **196**, 129–54.

Nowakowski, R. S. & Wahlsten, D. (1985a). Asymmetric development of the hippocampal region in the shaker short-tail (sst) mutant mouse. *Society for Neuroscience Abstracts*, **11**, 989.

(1985b). Anatomy and development of the hippocampus and dentate gyrus in the shaker short-tail (sst) mutant mouse. *Anatomical Record*, **211**, 140A.

O'Leary, D. D. (1987). Remodeling of early projections through the selective elimination of neurons and long axon collaterals. *CIBA Foundation Symposium*, **126**, 113–42.

O'Leary, D. D. & Stanfield, B. B. (1985). Occipital cortical neurons with transient pyramidal tract axons extend and maintain collaterals to subcortical but not intracortical targets. *Brain Research*, **336**, 326–33.

Oppenheim, R. W. (1981). Neuronal cell death and some related regressive phenomena during neurogenesis: A selective historical review and progress report. In W. M. Cowan (Ed.), *Studies in Developmental Neurobiology* (pp. 74–133). New York: Oxford University Press.

Otake, M. & Schull, W. J. (1984). *In utero* exposure to A-bomb radiation and mental retardation: a reassessment. *British Journal of Radiology*, **57**, 409–14.

Pearlman, A. L. (1985). The visual cortex of the normal mouse and reeler mutant. In E. G. Jones & A. A. Peters (Eds), *The Cerebral Cortex* (pp. 1–18). New York: Plenum Press.

Purves, D. & Hadley, R. D. (1985). Changes in the dendritic branching of adult mammalian neurons revealed by repeated imaging *in situ*. *Nature, London*, **315**, 404–6.

Purves, D. & Lichtman, J. W. (1985). *Principles of Neural Development*. Sunderland, Massachusetts: Sinauer.

Purves, D., Snider, W. D. & Voyvodic, J. T. (1988). Trophic regulation of nerve cell morphology and innervation in the autonomic nervous system. *Nature, London*, **336**, 123–8.

Purves, D., Voyvodic, J. T., Magrassi, L. & Yawo, H. (1987). Nerve terminal remodeling visualized in living mice by repeated examination of the same neuron. *Science*, **238**, 1122–6.

Rakic, P. (1971). Neuron–glia relationship during granule cell migration in developing cerebellar cortex: A Golgi and electron microscopic study in Macacus rhesus. *Journal of Comparative Neurology*, **141**, 283–312.

(1972). Mode of migration to the superficial layers of fetal monkey neocortex. *Journal of Comparative Neurology*, **145**, 61–83.

(1975a). Cell migration and neuronal ectopias in the brain. *Birth Defects: Original Article Series*, **11**(7), 95–129.

(1975b). Timing of major ontogenetic events in the visual cortex of the rhesus monkey. In *Brain Mechanisms in Mental Retardation* (pp. 3–40). New York: Academic Press.

(1977). Genesis of the dorsal lateral geniculate nucleus in the rhesus monkey:

Site and time of origin, kinetics of proliferation, routes of migration and pattern of distribution of neurons. *Journal of Comparative Neurology*, **176**, 23–52.

(1978). Neuronal migration and contact guidance in the primate telencephalon. *Postgraduate Medical Journal*, **54**, 25–40.

(1982). Early developmental events: Cell lineages, acquisition of neuronal positions, and areal and laminar development. *Neuroscience Research Progress Bulletin*, **20**, 439–51.

(1985). Limits of neurogenesis in primates. *Science*, **227**, 1054–6.

(1988). Specification of cerebral cortical areas. *Science*, **241**, 170.

Rakic, P., Bourgeois, J.-P., Eckenhoff, M. F., Zecevic, N. & Goldman-Rakic, P. S. (1986). Concurrent overproduction of synapses in diverse regions of the primate cerebral cortex. *Science*, **232**, 232–5.

Rakic, P. & Goldman-Rakic, P. S. (1982). The development and modifiability of the cerebral cortex: Overview. *Neuroscience Research Progress Bulletin*, **20**, 433–8.

Rakic, P. & Nowakowski, R. S. (1981). The time of origin of neurons in the hippocampal region of the rhesus monkey. *Journal of Comparative Neurology*, **196**, 99–128.

Rakic, P. & Riley, K. P. (1983). Regulation of axon number in primate optic nerve by prenatal binocular competition. *Nature*, **305**, 135–7.

Rakic, P., Stensaas, L. J., Sayre, E. P. & Sidman, R. L. (1974). Computer-aided three-dimensional reconstruction and quantitative analysis of cells from serial electron microscopic montages of foetal monkey brain. *Nature, London*, **250**, 31–4.

Richardson, E. P., Jr (1982). Myelination in the human central nervous system. In W. Haymaker & R. D. Adams (Eds.), *Histology and Histopathology of the Nervous System*, (vol. I, pp. 146–73). Springfield: Thomas.

Richman, D. P., Stewart, R. M., Hutchinson, J. W. & Caviness, V. S., Jr (1975). Mechanical model of brain convolutional development. *Science*, **189**, 18–21.

Schmidt, J. T. (1985a). Selective stabilization of retinotectal synapses by an activity-dependent mechanism. *Federation Proceedings*, **44**, 2767–72.

(1985b). Activity-dependent synaptic stabilization in development and learning: How similar the mechanisms? *Cellular and Molecular Neurobiology*, **5**, 1–3.

Schmidt, J. T. & Tieman, S. B. (1985). Eye-specific segregation of optic afferents in mammals, fish, and frogs: The role of activity. *Cellular and Molecular Neurobiology*, **5**, 5–34.

Segraves, M. A. & Innocenti, G. M. (1985). Comparison of the distributions of ipsilaterally and contralaterally projecting corticocortical neurons in cat visual cortex using two fluorescent tracers. *The Journal of Neuroscience*, **5**, 2107–18.

Sidman, R. L. (1961). Histogenesis of mouse retina studied with thymidine–³H. In G. Smelser (Ed.), *Structure of the Eye* (pp. 487–506). New York: Academic Press.

Sidman, R. L. & Rakic, P. (1973). Neuronal migration with special reference to developing human brain: A review. *Brain Research*, **62**, 1–35.

Smart, I. H. M. & McSherry, G. M. (1982). Growth patterns in the lateral wall of the mouse telencephalon: II. Histological changes during and subsequent to the period of isocortical neuron production. *Journal of Anatomy*, **134**, 415–42.

Stanfield, B. B. & O'Leary, D. D. (1985a). Fetal occipital cortical neurons transplanted to the rostral cortex can extend and maintain a pyramidal tract axon. *Nature, London*, **313**, 135–7.

(1985b). The transient corticospinal projection from the occipital cortex during the postnatal development of the rat. *Journal of Comparative Neurology*, **238**, 236–48.

Taber-Pierce, E. (1972). Time of origin of neurons in the brain stem of the mouse. *Progress in Brain Research*, **40**, 53–66.

Temple, S. & Raff, M. C. (1986). Clonal analysis of oligodendrocyte development in culture: Evidence for a developmental clock that counts cell divisions. *Cell*, **44**, 773–9.

Toulouse, G., Dehanes, S. & Changeux, J. P. (1986). Spin glass model of learning by selection. *Proceedings of the National Academy of Sciences, USA*, **83**, 1695–8.

Walsh, C., Polley, E. H., Hickey, T. L. & Guillery, R. W. (1983). Generation of cat retinal ganglion cells in relation to central pathways. *Nature, London*, **302**, 611–14.

Wiesel, T. N. (1982). Postnatal development of the visual cortex and the influence of environment. *Nature, London*, **299**, 583–91.

Wyss, J. M. & Sripanidkulchai, B. (1985). The development of Ammon's horn and the fascia dentata in the cat: A [^{3}H]thymidine analysis. *Developmental Brain Research*, **18**, 185–98.

Zimmerman, R. A., Bilaniuk, L. T. & Grossman, R. I. (1983). Computed tomography in migratory disorders of human brain development. *Neuroradiology*, **25**, 257–63.

3

The development of primate neocortex – an overview

E. G. JONES

University of California, Irvine

Introduction

The cerebral cortex of primates shows a highly ordered but complex pattern of connectivity, lamination and cytoarchitecture. Such complexity arises from an orderly sequence of developmental events that commences with a relatively simple pattern of cellular proliferation and migration and proceeds to connection-formation, the establishment of cytoarchitectonic boundaries, and the genesis of definitive neuronal phenotypes. These critical events in mammalian neocortical development have been the subject of much recent research, and the potential for perturbations at critical stages to induce disorders of subsequent cortical organization is being revealed.

Fundamental cortical structure

The primate cerebral cortex is divided into a number of cytoarchitectonic fields, each distinguished with greater or lesser clarity from its neighbors by differences in cell size, shape and packing density which determine the variations in the cortical layers. In some areas, certain subregions acquire separate cytoarchitectural identities. The callosally connected part of the human and monkey primary visual area (Shoumura, 1974; Shoumura, Ando & Kato, 1975; Glickstein & Whitteridge, 1976) is a case in point. Here, the part of area 17 adjoining area 18 possesses a denser concentration of large pyramidal cells in deep layer III than the remainder of the area.

The traditional cytoarchitectonicist's view is that virtually every cortical area differs from its fellows. However, recent quantitative studies of a number of cytoarchitectonic areas in several species suggest a considerable degree of homogeneity from area to area (Rockel, Hiorns & Powell, 1974, 1980; Beaulieu & Colonnier, 1983, 1985, 1989; Hendry et al., 1987a).

Rockell, Hiorns & Powell (1980) discovered that there was a remarkable uniformity in cell number per 30μm-wide column extending through the thickness of the cortex from pia mater to white matter, not only from area to area of single species but also across species. In the mouse the number of cells per column did not differ greatly from that in the somewhat thicker cortex of primates. Area 17 of primates was the only area showing a significant difference from all other areas. There, the cell number per column was more than double that in columns in other areas of primates and approximately double that of columns in the visual areas of nonprimates. Differences in cortical thickness across species are not great, the average cortical thickness in a mouse being approximately 1–1.5 mm and that of a human 4–5 mm. Hence, for all cortical areas except the primary visual area of primates, changes in cortical thickness per unit area are probably achieved to a large extent by modifying the neuropil and not by changing significantly the number of neurons per column. Moreover, it would appear that the vast expansion of the cortex in the evolution of the primate brain has occurred by the addition of more unitary, column-like groupings of cells.

The studies of Colonnier and his associates on the cat are not in complete agreement with that of Rockel et al., for in their hands the motor area shows fewer cells per unit column than the visual and somatic sensory areas. The studies of Hendry et al. (1987a) on ten areas of monkey cortex tend to support them, however. These studies also demonstrated the contribution of the subpopulation of cortical neurons that expressed immunoreactivity for the inhibitory transmitter, gamma aminobutyric acid (GABA), to the total (Table 3.1). The number of GABA neurons per arbitrary 50-μm-wide column follows a similar pattern of consistency, the percentage being about 25% for most areas. Area 17 is the exception. There, despite a large increase in GABA neuron numbers, the GABA cell population falls to about 20% on account of the twofold increase in total neuron number (see also Schwartz, Zheng & Goldman-Rakic, 1988).

These data argue for a fundamental similarity in neuronal numbers and proportions of particular neuronal types from area to area of the primate cortex. Area 17, although different from other areas, shows a consistent difference across primate species. Hence, the development of cytoarchitectonic areas in the cortex, if based upon the assembly of modular, column-like groupings of neurons, is likely to be based upon the assembly of groupings that do not differ greatly from one another numerically. The consistency in the proportion of GABA neurons per radial unit in the adult further suggests

Table 3.1. *Mean number (±SD) of GABA-immunoreactive neurons and of all neurons in 50-μm-wide columns through the thickness of cortical areas 4, 3b, 1–2, 5, 7, 18 and 17 in five different monkeys.*

Area	CM 181			CM 187		
	GABA	Total	%	GABA	Total	%
4	39.0±2.9	158.9±16.1	24.5±2.0	39.4±2.7	159.4±16.3	24.5±1.3
3b	39.9±2.8	152.7±11.9	26.1±1.7	32.1±5.9	154.9±11.7	20.6±1.2
1–2	40.1±2.6	154.8±14.2	25.9±1.8	38.4±4.0	157.9±16.1	24.4±2.1
5	40.4±2.2	163.1±10.6	24.7±2.3	39.2±2.0	160.6±14.1	24.4±1.9
7	38.4±2.9	158.2±9.4	24.1±1.6	40.7±3.7	158.8±14.8	25.1±1.4
18	38.1±2.9	157.3±10.1	24.4±2.1	38.6±3.6	157.9±15.0	24.7±2.1
17	59.1±5.7	315.7±19.4	18.7±2.1	58.2±5.7	309.9±22.7	19.2±2.0

Area	CM 183			CM 189		
	GABA	Total	%	GABA	Total	%
4	40.4±3.9	161.7±15.3	25.0±1.7	39.4±2.4	161.6±17.0	24.3±2.1
3b	33.1±5.0	157.9±12.2	21.0±2.1	40.1±3.0	156.5±12.7	25.6±2.3
1–2	38.0±3.3	154.3±11.6	24.6±2.3	38.4±3.3	158.8±11.9	24.0±1.9
5	39.1±2.7	155.3±9.4	25.2±1.8	38.5±3.4	155.1±12.0	24.9±2.0
7	39.9±2.9	157.6±11.8	25.3±1.3	40.4±2.4	160.1±16.5	25.2±2.4
18	38.4±3.9	152.0±9.1	25.3±1.6	38.1±2.9	157.5±17.5	24.2±1.7
17	61.1±4.7	309.8±17.1	19.6±1.5	59.1±5.7	321.3±23.6	18.5±2.2

Table 3.1. (cont.)

CM 184

Area	GABA	Total	%
4	40.7±3.4	157.1±15.5	25.2±1.1
3b	32.9±5.7	160.4±11.0	20.2±1.9
1–2	40.1±3.1	154.9±9.7	25.1±1.7
5	40.4±2.0	158.1±13.0	24.9±1.3
7	40.7±2.8	159.9±11.7	24.3±2.0
18	40.8±5.0	158.4±16.2	24.7±1.8
17	60.3±5.3	319.6±21.4	19.1±1.0

Counts of GABA-positive neurons and of all neurons were made at a magnification of 1250 from adjacent sections, and the percentages of GABA cells were calculated from the quotient of the 2 values.
Source: Hendry et al. (1987).

that the relative percentages of cells of different types could also be maintained in each hypothetical modular grouping.

The neocortex develops in a manner that has been interpreted as indicative of a repeating radial pattern of neurons (Rakic, 1988). Young neurons are generated in the ventricular or subventricular zones of the neuroepithelium and migrate into the overlying cortical plate by following the processes of radial glial cells (Rakic, 1972). Young neurons are commonly lined up in columns along the radial glial processes, and resemble the sort of clone that would be expected to arise from a single precursor cell in the neuroepithelium. This, in turn, could lead to the formation of a basic columnar unit of cortical architecture (Rakic & Goldman-Rakic, 1982; Mountcastle, 1978; Rakic, 1988). Hence, the size of a cortical area might be governed by the number of radial units allocated to it in the neuroepithelium. Studies involving retrovirus infection of cortical precursor cells should enable workers to determine whether a clonal pattern can account for the columnarity of the cortex. However, results to date have been variously interpreted as either supporting or negating a columnar, developmental pattern (Luskin, Pearlman & Sanes, 1988; Price & Thurlow, 1988; Walsh & Cepko, 1988). It is obvious, however, that interference with the processes of neuronal proliferation and migration could have disastrous consequences for the patterns of cytoarchitectonic order and the sizes of cytoarchitectonic fields in the adult primate cortex. These, in turn, will have further consequences for the connections made between cortical areas and the rest of the brain, for connectivity and cytoarchitecture are inextricably linked.

The establishment of afferent innervation

The cytoarchitectonic delineation of the cerebral cortex is closely correlated with afferent, efferent and intrinsic connectivity. The fiber terminations of many afferent systems are limited by architectonic borders and certain populations of cells projecting to a particular target are found in some cortical areas but not in others. During development, there appears to be a complex interplay between intrinsic factors and afferent connectivity in the establishment of the cytoarchitectonic and functional fields of the neocortex.

Cytoarchitectonic field structure is not discernible when a cortical plate first appears in the telencephalic wall. However, areas could still be predetermined in the neuroepithelium. It appears that only a restricted zone of proliferation in the ventricular lining contributes cells to a particular field (Rakic, 1974). Areal borders become clearly evident as the cortical plate disappears relatively early in development, and lamination becomes established in sequential order from deep to superficial.

Thalamic and callosal axons arrive relatively early in the vicinity of the developing sensory–motor and visual areas of the cortex, but they undergo a relatively protracted waiting period in the underlying white matter (intermediate zone) and only commence invading the cortex as the cortical plate is disappearing and cortical laminae and cytoarchitectonic borders are becoming established (Wise and Jones, 1976, 1978; Rakic, 1988; Lund & Mustari, 1977; Wise, Hendry & Jones, 1977; Shatz & Luskin, 1986). In monkeys, the border between areas 17 and 18, and to a large extent the laminar structure of area 17, can be discerned before the invasion of the cortex by geniculocortical afferents around day 110 of gestation (Rakic, 1988). The border between areas 3a and 4 is readily discernible before day 110, afferent and efferent connectivity arriving at about the same time (Killackey & Chalupa, 1986; Huntley, Jones & DeBlas, 1990). It is difficult to see that the two major afferent systems could play an inducing role in setting up architectonic field borders because they arrive as border formation is commencing and many aspects of cortical field structure will still develop if thalamic and callosal fibers are removed before they enter the cortex (Wise & Jones, 1978). However, there is the growing possibility of interactions with migrating cells growing through the fibers as they lie in the intermediate zone beneath the cortex (see below).

Intra-areal remodeling occurs as the extrinsic innervation becomes established. Area 4 of the monkey fetus possesses a clearly distinct granular layer IV up to birth but becomes agranular as postnatal development proceeds (Huntley et al., 1990). Similarly, the lamination that distinguishes areas 3a, 3b, 1 and 2 in the postcentral gyrus only becomes clear-cut as afferent innervation develops. The cytochrome oxidase containing periodicities visible in layer III of area 17 in the monkey only become detectable late in fetal life (Horton & Hedley-Whyte, 1984). These are indications of subareal architecture crystallizing out as afferent connectivity is being established. Similar remodeling under the influence of afferent innervation occurs in the somatic sensory cortex of rodents (Van der Loos & Woolsey, 1973; Killackey, Ivy & Cunningham, 1978) indicating the influence of the periphery not necessarily as a determinant of architectonic borders but of subareal structure.

In experiments in monkeys from which both eyes had been removed during intrauterine life, the area 17/18 border was still visible postnatally but area 17 was reduced in size (Rakic, 1988; Dehay et al., 1989). It is possible, therefore, that a further major feature determined by interactions with afferent fibers is cortical field size.

The influence of the subplate

It is possible that afferent fibers exert a remote influence on cortical development by interacting with migrating cells before the arrival of either fibers or cells in the cortex. Afferent fibers innervating a cortical area arise in the thalamus and in the ipsi- and contralateral cortex as well as among the monoamine and cholinergic cell groups of the brainstem or basal forebrain (Fig. 3.1). These latter appear to colonize the cortex first (Schlumpf, Shoemaker & Bloom, 1980; Caviness & Korde, 1981; Kristt & Molliver, 1976; Verney et al., 1982; Marin-Padilla, 1984, 1988) and seem to be present among the cells that migrate first to the wall of the telencephalon. This population of earliest-generated cells, appearing before E70 in monkeys, is subsequently split into two strata, superficial and deep, by the arrival of later waves of cells that form the cortical plate. The two strata become the marginal zone or primitive layer I, and a transient region called the subplate in which arriving afferent fibers accumulate and through which all cells destined for the cortical plate must migrate. The cortical plate gives rise to layers II–VI of the cortex.

In monkeys, arriving thalamocortical axons start to accumulate in the subplate part of the intermediate zone beneath the cortical plate in the middle of gestation (approximately E80), and invade the cortex subsequent to E110, achieving their final laminar pattern of distribution by about E124–144 (Rakic, 1988). Fiber ingrowth appears to be initially somewhat diffuse, with columnar and laminar distribution patterns appearing at or about the time the definitive laminar distribution is established. In the monkey visual system, the final columnar distribution is achieved only under the influence of normal postnatal visual experience (Hubel, Wiesel & LeVay, 1977; Le Vay, Wiesel & Hubel, 1980).

While accumulating in the subplate zone, thalamocortical, corticocortical and commissural fibers lie among the population of subplate neurons. Growing through them, en route to the overlying cortex, are the waves of cell migrations destined to form the middle and superficial layers of the cortex in which the afferent fibers will eventually terminate. The extent to which the accumulating fibers, the subplate cells and the migrating young cortical cells recognize one another, and whether information is exchanged between them, is currently unknown. An exchange of signals that could be required for subsequent recognition of target cells by the fibers and synapse formation in the cortex is a possibility that has not been verified. Synapse-like structures, certain transmitter receptors, and synaptic vesicle antigens are demonstrable in the subplate region (and in layer I) before their appearance in the cortical plate (Kristt & Molliver, 1976; Chun & Shatz, 1988; Huntley et al., 1990).

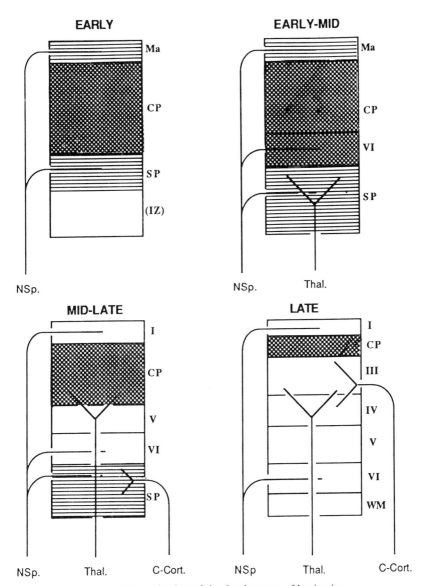

Figure 3.1. Schematic view of the development of lamination and afferent innervation in the cerebral cortex at early, early-mid, mid-late and late phases of gestation. Nonspecific afferents (NSp.) colonize the marginal (Ma) and subplate (SP) zones first and later invade deeper layers of cortex as layer VI develops out of the cortical plate (CP). Thalamic (Thal.), followed by commissural and associational (C-Cort.) afferents, accumulate in the subplate and invade the cortex as the other layers emerge from the cortical plate. WM, white matter; IZ, intraventricular zone.

These suggest the presence of a synaptic zone in the subplate zone. Immunoreactivity for the synaptic vesicle antigens and receptors disappears from the subplate as fibers invade the cortex, and it now appears in the cortex proper. The subplate cells may also play an important role in the guidance of cortical efferent fibers to their targets (McConnell, Ghosh & Shatz, 1989).

Many of the corticocortical and callosal fibers may be inappropriate for the overlying area and may never enter the cortex (Clarke & Innocenti, 1986). Those that do so tend to invade the overlying cortex a short time after the thalamic fibers. The initial ingrowth of these other two fiber systems is usually reported as diffuse (Wise & Jones, 1976, 1978; Rakic, 1988) with a later redistribution of the fibers into the patchy, dysjunctive distribution patterns of corticocortical and callosal fibers seen in many cortical areas in the adult. This suggests interactions with the thalamocortical fibers as they are setting up their definitive patterns of distribution.

The nature of the interactions between afferent fibers in the subplate region and in the maturing cortex is not completely known. Interference with one set of afferents, for example the visual thalamocortical system by removal of the eyes, may lead to changes in the distribution of commissural fiber terminations so that the diffuse pattern of the immature cortex is retained (Innocenti & Frost, 1979; Cusick & Lund, 1982; Olavarria & van Sluyters, 1985). The disruptions of the visual pathway found in the Siamese cat (Hubel & Wiesel, 1977; Guillery & Kaas, 1971; Shatz, 1977a,b), and those resulting from the induction of a strabismus in normal infant cats (Lund, Mitchell & Henry, 1978; Innocenti & Frost, 1979), lead to changes in the patterns of retinotopic organization and of callosal fiber distribution that suggest the normal occurrence of developmental interactions between thalamic and callosal axons. It is probable that corticocortical and callosal fibers under conditions of perturbed afferent input survive in inappropriate regions by gaining an advantage over thalamocortical fibers. They are further reflections of the important role played by ordered patterns of afferent activity in determining the later phases of cortical development during which the normal patterns of afferent connectivity are being established.

Activity-dependent regulation of cortical structure

Afferent activity is essential for the normal maturation of neuronal function in the visual cortex of primates (reviewed in Hubel & Wiesel, 1977; Blakemore, Garey & Vital-Durand, 1978; Movshon & Van Sluyters, 1981), and it is likely that similar conditions will operate in other sensory areas. During a critical early period of postnatal development (3–4 months in the macaque monkey), perturbations of visual experience can seriously compromise the establishment of normal cortical cell physiology. Many such perturbations lead also to morphological effects. Removal of one eye, deactivation of one retina by injections of tetrodotoxin, or the reduction by eyelid suture of patterned stimuli entering one eye during the critical period, results in a more extensive distribution of the terminal ramifications of thalamocortical fibers related to the normal eye and a reciprocal less extensive distribution of those related to the perturbed eye (Hubel *et al.*, 1977; LeVay *et al.*, 1980). In the course of normal visual cortex development, right-eye and left-eye thalamocortical fibers withdraw from substantially overlapping territories into their own ocular dominance domains. This is probably the result of competitive interactions in which each has an equal advantage. It is asynchrony in the inputs from the two eyes that seems primarily to contribute to this effect for, in the presence of monocular deprivation by tetrodotoxin injection in cats during the critical period, the normal columnar pattern of development can still be induced by asynchronous electrical stimulation of the two optic nerves but prevented by synchronous stimulation of the two nerves (Stryker & Harris, 1986; Stryker & Strickland, 1984). It is probably the spontaneous activity of the retina that initiates the segregation of ocular dominance columns *in utero* and, even when reared in the dark, animals show segregation of such columns.

The onset of normal neural activity is thus a powerful epigenetic influence on subsequent establishment of fine topographic order in the mammalian cerebral cortex. As such, interference with the normal onset of activity may have profound effects on adult cortical structure and function.

Activity-dependent changes in cortical maps

As indicated above, the development of normal cortical function requires sensory experience. But the maintenance of cortical topographic organization throughout life also appears to depend on sensory activity. In the somatic sensory areas of several species, particularly primates (Merzenich *et al.*, 1983*a*,*b*, 1984, 1988; Kelahan & Doetsch, 1984; McKinley & Kruger, 1988), following removal of a portion of the receptive periphery, such as a finger, previously silent representations of adjacent peripheral regions, such as parts of adjacent fingers, are revealed within the part of the map that would be expected to be silenced. Excessive stimulation of a normal finger may also lead to the expansion of that finger's cortical representation at the expense of that of others. These effects occur so rapidly that it is unlikely that they are the result of axon sprouting and new synapse formation. Instead, they suggest the uncovering or strengthening of connections that are normally suppressed under the conditions of the experiments.

49

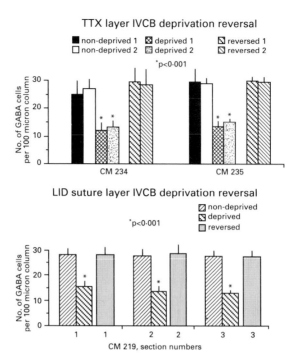

Figure 3.2. Number of GABA-immunoreactive neurons in 100 μm wide columns through layer IVCB of the visual cortex of two monkeys subjected to monocular visual deprivation by tetrodotoxin (TTX) injection or eyelid suture. Left pairs in each trio of bar graphs show reduction in stainable cells in deprived eye columns in comparison with normal eye columns, in a biopsy from the cortex. Right bar of each trio shows return to normal numbers after a period of renewed binocular visual exposure. (From Hendry and Jones, 1988.)

Two bases for these rapid, activity-dependent changes in cortical maps in the adult primate seem likely to be found, first, in the presence of terminations of single thalamocortical axons that are normally not revealed in conventional extracellular mapping (Snow *et al.*, 1988), and, second, in the activity-dependent regulation of transmitter production, particularly of GABA, in cortical neurons (Hendry & Jones, 1986, 1988).

GABA normally exerts a powerful influence on cortical neurons (Dykes *et al.*, 1984; Alloway & Burton, 1986; Sillito, 1975, 1979; Sillito, Kemp & Blakemore, 1981). In normal animals, when GABA receptors are selectively blocked, elements of receptive field structure are revealed that indicate normally suppressed inputs from other parts of the receptive periphery. In the cerebral cortex of normal adult monkeys, production of the enzyme that is involved in GABA synthesis, glutamic acid decarboxylase (GAD), is activity-dependent. Experimentally-induced blockade of action potentials in the optic nerve leads within four days to a 50% reduction in cells immunoreactive for GAD and GABA in the relevant eye dominance columns of the visual cortex. This effect is reversed by restoration of binocular vision (Hendry & Jones, 1986, 1988) (Fig. 3.2). Similar activity-dependent regulation of GABA undoubtedly occurs in other areas of the primate cortex, and should have a profound influence on the receptive fields of single neurons and upon the maps of the external world.

Similar effects are likely to play a profound role in the cortex during its development and maturation. As development proceeds and neuronal function is brought under the influence of afferent activity, the neurotransmitter plasticity revealed in the adult is likely to be a major determinant of connectional stabilization and the development of normal cortical representations.

Neurotransmitter effects on neocortical plasticity

Noradrenaline and acetylcholine

Experience-dependent modifications of the visual cortex during a critical developmental period were mentioned above. Cats, monocularly deprived for the first three months of life, never acquire normal vision with the deprived eye and this is associated with a radical shift in the responsivity of cells in the visual cortex in the direction of the nondeprived eye (Dews & Wiesel, 1970; Wiesel & Hubel, 1965; reviewed in Sherman & Spear, 1982, and Movshon & Van Sĺuyters, 1981). In monkeys, the critical period for some effects seems to extend into the first year of life (Blakemore et al., 1978).

The large number of studies that have been conducted on the plasticity of the maturing visual cortex, especially in cats, strongly indicates that the effect is dependent upon the weakening and strengthening of synaptic inputs to cortical neurons and that it depends upon the presence of a behavioral context. Ocular dominance changes, for example, do not occur if a monocularly deprived kitten is paralyzed and anesthetized (Freeman & Bonds, 1979; Buisseret, Gary-Bobo & Imbert, 1978; Rauschecker & Singer, 1982). Changes in synaptic efficiency and the permissive role of behavioral context suggest that afferent systems that exert a modulatory effect over cortical synapses, and afferent systems that control behavioral state, could be critically involved. The brainstem afferent systems that are involved in state-dependent behavior innervate the cortex diffusely and release transmitters such as noradrenaline and acetylcholine, which seem to have a modulatory effect upon cortical synapses (Videen, Daw & Rader, 1984; Singer, 1988). Hence, the coincidence of increased inputs from one eye and facilitatory effects from the nonspecific afferent systems may be critical in increasing the efficacy of synapses driven by that eye at the expense of synapses driven by the deprived eye. Indeed, stimulation of the mesencephalic reticular formation can, when combined with monocular stimulation, lead to a shift in ocular dominance even in paralyzed kittens (Rauschecker & Singer, 1982).

The neurotransmitter agents released by the diffusely distributed brain-stem and basal forebrain pathways can influence visual cortical plasticity in cats under certain conditions. Local infusion of 6–hydroxydopamine, or other agents that deplete noradrenaline in the cortex of cats during the critical period, is effective in preventing the expected ocular dominance shift of monocular deprivation (Kasamatsu, Pettigrew & Ary, 1979; Daw et al., 1983, 1984, 1985 a,b; Adrien et al., 1985; Bear et al., 1983). If the locus cœruleus and the cholinergic pathways arising in the basal forebrain are destroyed so as to deplete both noradrenaline and aceylcholine in the cortex, the ocular dominance shift caused by monocular deprivation is also prevented, but destruction of either system alone is ineffective. This implies that the cholinergic and noradrenergic afferent systems interact in the selective synaptic stabilization that appears to underlie experience-dependent cortical plasticity.

Other transmitters

Both the inhibitory transmitter, GABA, and an excitatory acidic amino acid transmitter acting as the N–methyl–D–aspartate (NMDA) receptor have also been implicated in experience-dependent plasticity of the maturing visual cortex of cats. A small number of visual cortical cells that become responsive only to the normal eye after monocular deprivation in the critical period retain a suppressed deprived-eye input which can be demonstrated under the influence of the GABA antagonist, bicuculline (Sillito et al., 1981). This suggests that GABA-mediated inhibition is enhanced in deprived eye columns. Blockade of the NMDA receptor by infusion of the antagonist, aminophosphonovalerate (APV), into the visual cortex of kittens in the critical period prevents the ocular dominance shift normally induced by monocular deprivation. APV also prevents (in part) the reversal of the shift that can be induced if, during the critical period, a lid-sutured eye is opened and the formerly nondeprived eye closed (Bode-Gruel & Singer, 1989). Thus, other neurotransmitter systems additional to those of the nonspecific afferent systems may exert a permissive effect on the plasticity of synaptic stabilization that exists during the critical period. Because afferent activity regulates several neurotransmitter and neuropeptide systems in the adult cortex (see Part VI), this neurotransmitter-dependent modulation of developing cortical synapses is likely to depend upon a complex interplay of activity arriving in all cortical afferent systems.

Neurotransmitter and neuropeptide expression in developing cortical neurons

During the normal development of the monkey cortex, changes occur over time in the appearance and distribution of cortical neurons exhibiting immunoreactivity for particular neurotransmitters, their receptors and neuropeptides (Huntley et al., 1988a,b) (Fig. 3.3). Similar changes have been more thoroughly documented in other species (see Shaw et al., 1984, 1986). In the visual and sensory–motor cortex of the monkey, the cytoarchitecture is virtually adult-like by the end of the second third of gestation, but the distributions of GABA and peptide cells continue to change. Substantial populations of tachykinin cells, for example, are found early in layer V of the visual cortex but then decline and increase in layer IVC. Certain populations, notably those showing immunoreactivity for choline acetyltransferase or proenkephalin, are not found in adults, and have only a transient appearance in the developing cortex (Hendry et al. 1987b; Huntley et al., 1988a). Especially evident at the early stages are substantial populations of neurons immunoreactive for neuropeptide Y, somatostatin, proenkephalin and GABA in the subplate beneath the developing cortex (Fig. 3.3). Although never completely disappearing, their numbers decline as development proceeds, probably as the result of selective cell death (Chun & Shatz, 1989). The populations of cortical neurons detectable by immunocytochemistry become evident at about the time that thalamocortical fibers commence entering the cortex, and the major changes in their numbers and distribution occur as cortical innervation is being established.

The precise role of any particular cortical transmitter or neuropeptide in the early development of the cerebral cortex is unknown. It is clear, however, that several neurotransmitters affect the plasticity and stabilization of the cortex during the later, critical periods. Transmitter expression in the mature cortex is activity-dependent and in the developing cortex the maturation of neurotransmitter- and neuropeptide-expressing cells is coincident with the arrival of afferent fibers, suggesting that it too depends on afferent activity. But the onset of transmitter function may itself have inductive effects. There is growing evidence from non-mammalian and *in-vitro* systems that not only neural activity but associated influences mediated by neurotransmitters and possibly neuropeptides can have a profound effect on neural morphogenesis

NPY

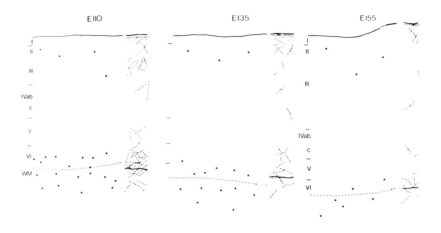

GABA

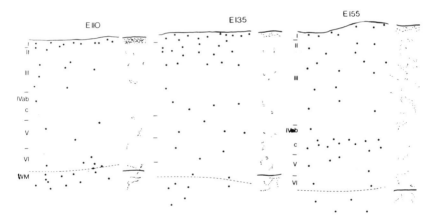

Figure 3.3. Upper: changes in the distribution of neuropeptide-immunoreactive cells and fibers in the visual cortex of monkey fetuses at the gestation ages indicated. Lower: changes in the GABA-immunoreactive population. (From Huntley *et al.*, 1988a.)

54

and connection formation (Lipton & Kater, 1989). Thus, the interplay of neuronal activity, gene expression for transmitters, peptides and their receptors, and interactions between these are likely to play major roles in the early establishment of patterns of cortical connectivity, and perturbations at any point may have substantial later effects.

The establishment of efferent innervation

Axon outgrowth from cortical neurons occurs early and starts to occur even before a neuron has completed its migration to the cortical plate (Schreyer & Jones, 1982; Schwartz, Zheng & Goldman-Rakic, 1988). The axons growing out from the cortical efferent neurons display a high degree of target specificity, and those growing from cells destined for a particular layer invariably seem to reach targets appropriate for that layer even if the migration of the parent cells is perturbed or obstructed (Floeter & Jones, 1985; Jones, Valentino & Fleshman, 1982; Yurkewicz et al., 1984; McConnell, 1985).

Although laminar-specified cells make few or no mistakes in terms of the general targets to which they send axons, the cells early on have the capacity to grow axon branches to distant sites to which they do not normally project in the adult. In neonatal rats, for example, layer V cells with axons projecting to the brainstem and spinal cord are found throughout far greater extents of neocortex than they occupy in the adult (O'Leary & Stanfield, 1985, 1986; Schreyer & Jones, 1988b). In neonatal cats, corticocortical axons arising in the auditory cortex pass towards the visual areas, a pathway that does not exist in the adult (Innocenti, Clark & Kraftsik, 1986). In many species, callosal axons pass towards cortical areas that are inappropriate for them or normally devoid of commissural connections (Innocenti, 1981; Innocenti & Caminiti, 1980; Chalupa & Killackey, 1989; Killackey & Chalupa, 1986; Dehay et al., 1986, 1988). In the further course of development, axon collaterals arising from inappropriately sited cells are pruned, leaving the parent cell intact with its 'appropriate' axon (O'Leary & Stanfield, 1986; Innocenti et al., 1986; Chalupa & Killackey, 1989). Even within appropriately targeted axonal systems, however, many axons appear to be lost.

There is a substantially greater number of cortical efferent axons growing towards a particular target in the developing brain than in the tracts of the mature brain and spinal cord. In the corpus callosum of monkeys and cats 70% of the axons are reported to disappear between birth and adulthood (Berbel & Innocenti, 1988). In the corticospinal tract of rats (Schreyer & Jones, 1988b; Gorgels et al., 1989) and the pyramidal tract of hamsters (Reh & Kalil, 1981, 1982), corresponding losses of axons occur in the later phases of development. The factors that influence this loss are incompletely known but probably involve the whole range of developmentally-regulated events that includes axon–substrate interactions in axon guidance and target finding, target recognition and competition for synaptic space at the target site. All are presumably points at which perturbations can occur.

Development of the neuropil

In the cerebral cortex of fetal mammals, cell density is particularly high. Although the numerical density of cells has not been quantified in the primate cerebral cortex at the critical prenatal stages of development, between birth and six months of age neuronal density in the macaque monkey visual cortex decreases by approximately 30% without a corresponding loss in neuronal numbers (O'Kusky & Colonnier, 1982a,b). Prior to birth, a considerable degree of cell death has probably occurred.

The neuropil of the postnatal cortex expands as dendrites and axons grow and branch and as synapses are formed on the dendrites and somata. The density of synapses undergoes an enormous increase which continues well into postnatal life (O'Kusky & Colonnier, 1982b; Rakic et al., 1986). The density of synapses increases by 34% from birth to six months in the macaque monkey visual cortex, but then falls off and at maturity it is 95% less than at six months of age (O'Kusky & Colonnier, 1982a,b).

These synapses represent a combination derived from afferent fibers of all types, from axons of intrinsic neurons and from collateral axons of efferent neurons. The developmental regulation of their numbers appears to proceed independently of afferent influences since prenatal removal of the eyes in fetal monkeys does not influence the temporal sequence (Bourgeois, Jastreboff & Rakic, 1989). Postnatal visual experience, however, can have a profound influence on the ultimate density (Winfield, 1981).

The influences operating to reduce synaptic density as the cerebral cortex matures are undoubtedly those associated with the shaping of axonal distribution patterns and occurring under the influence of afferent activity. Competition for synaptic space and the stabilization of synapses with the onset of function (Changeux & Danchin, 1976) are probably the fundamental elements. These probably proceed under a large number of interrelated influences that will include the onset of afferent activity and the inductive effects of neurotransmitters and neuromodulators. The magnitude of the changes effected is likely to be under the influence of afferent activity during critical postnatal maturational periods.

Summary and conclusions

This survey has touched in a general way upon the major phases in the development of the primate cerebral cortex. It would be incorrect to assume, however, that primate neocortical development can be divided into self-contained epochs, for what emerges from a review of recent experimental studies is the clear evidence of a multidimensional process in which molecular–genetic and epigenetic influences interact in a place- and time-dependent manner and in which events occurring at one time may have consequences that are only manifested much later in the developmental process. Perturbations in place- and time-constrained developmental processes may therefore have major effects that may only reveal themselves much later. Perhaps the most powerful epigenetic influence on cortical development is the onset of afferent activity. But afferent influences are themselves multidimensional in the sense that different groups of afferent fibers enter the developing cortex at different times and may have inductive effects at an early stage and interact with each other at later stages in the stabilization of cortical connectivity. Afferent influences also supervene upon a pre-existing assembly of cortical neurons, the mechanisms of which assembly are still uncertain. It is clear, nevertheless, that all of the fundamental mechanisms of neuronal development that are being revealed in simpler systems are likely to be in action during the development of such a complicated structure as the primate neocortex. Many of these fundamental mechanisms, such as the activity-dependent regulation of sensory cortical maps and of transmitter and neuropeptide expression, appear to continue throughout the life of the animal. The consequences of perturbations in these fundamental mechanisms may, therefore, be far reaching and may only reveal themselves well after basic cortical development ends.

Acknowledgement

Supported by grant number MH44188 from the National Institute of Mental Health, United States Public Health Service.

References

Adrien, J., Blanc, G., Buisseret, P., Fregnac, Y., Gary-Bobo, E., Imbert, M., Tassin, J. P. & Trotter, Y. (1985). Noradrenaline and functional plasticity in kitten visual cortex: a re-examination. *Journal of Physiology (London)*, **367**, 73–98.

Alloway, K. D. & Burton, H. (1986). Bicuculline-induced alterations in neuronal responses to controlled tactile stimuli in the second somatosensory cortex of the cat: A microiontophoretic study. *Somatosensory Research*, **3**, 197–211.

57

Bear, M. F., Paradiso, M. A., Schwartz, M., Nelson, S. B., Carnes, K. M. & Daniels, J. D. (1983). Two methods of catecholamine depletion in kitten visual cortex yield different effects on plasticity. *Nature, London*, **302**, 245–57.

Bear, M. F. & Singer, W. (1986). Modulation of visual cortical plasticity by acetylcholine and noradrenaline. *Nature*, **320**, 172–6.

Beaulieu, C. & Colonnier, M. (1983). The number of neurons in the different laminae of the binocular and monocular regions of area 17 in the cat. *Journal of Comparative Neurology*, **217**, 337–44.

(1985). A comparison of the number of neurons in individual laminae of cortical areas 17, 18 and posteromedial suprasylvian (PMLS) area in the cat. *Brain Research*, **339**, 166–79.

(1989). Number of neurons in individual laminae of areas 3B, 4gamma, and 6alpha of the cat cerebral cortex: A comparison with major visual areas. *Journal of Comparative Neurology*, **279**, 228–34.

Berbel, P. & Innocenti, G. M. (1988). The development of the corpus callosum in cats: a light- and electron-microscopic study. *Journal of Comparative Neurology*, **276**, 132–56.

Blakemore, C., Garey, L. J. & Vital-Durand, F. (1978). The physiological effects of monocular deprivation and their reversal in monkey's visual cortex. *Journal of Physiology (London)*, **283**, 223–62.

Bode-Gruel, K. M. & Singer, W. (1989). The development of N–methyl–D–aspartate receptors in cat visual cortex. *Developmental Brain Research*, **466**, 197–204.

Bourgeois, J.-P., Jastreboff, P. J. & Rakic, P. (1989). Synaptogenesis in visual cortex of normal and preterm monkeys: Evidence for intrinsic regulation of synaptic overproduction. *Proceedings of the National Academy of Sciences, USA*, **86**, 4297–301.

Buisseret, P., Gary-Bobo, E. & Imbert, M. (1978). Ocular motility and recovery of orientational properties of visual cortical neurones in dark-reared kittens. *Nature*, London, **272**, 816–17.

Buisseret, P. & Imbert, P. (1976). Visual cortical cells: Their developmental properties in normal and dark-reared kittens. *Journal of Physiology (London)*, **255**, 511–25.

Caviness, V. S., Jr. & Korde, M. G. (1981). Monoaminergic afferents to the neocortex: A developmental histofluorescence study in normal and reeler mouse embryos. *Brain Research*, **209**, 1–9.

Chalupa, L. M. & Killackey, H. P. (1989). Process elimination underlies ontogenetic changes in the distribution of callosal projection neurons in the postcentral gyrus of the fetal rhesus monkey. *Proceedings of the National Academy of Sciences, USA*, **86**, 1076–9.

Changeux, J. P. & Danchin, A. (1976). Selective stabilisation of developing synapses as a mechanism for the specification of neuronal networks, *Nature, London*, **264**, 705–12.

Chun, J. J. M., Nakamura, M. J. & Shatz, C. J. (1987). Transient cells of the developing mammalian telencephalon are peptide immunoreactive neurons. *Nature, London*, **325**, 617–20.

Chun, J. J. M. & Shatz, C. J. (1988). A fibronectin-like molecule is present in the developing cat cerebral cortex and is correlated with subplate neurons. *Journal of Cell Biology*, **106**, 857–72.

(1989). Interstitial cells of the adult neocortical white matter are the remnant of the early-generated subplate neuron population. *Journal of Comparative Neurology*, **282**, 555–69.

Clarke, S. & Innocenti, G. M. (1986). Organization of immature intrahemispheric connections. *Journal of Comparative Neurology*, **251**, 1–22.

Cusick, C. G. & Lund, R. D. (1982). Modification of visual callosal projections in rats. *Journal of Comparative Neurology*, **212**, 385–98.

Daw, N. W., Rader, R. K., Robertson, T. W. & Ariel, M. (1983). Effects of 6–hydroxydopamine on visual deprivation in the kitten striate cortex. *The Journal of Neuroscience*, **3**, 907–14.

Daw, N. W., Robertson, T. W. & Rader, R. K. (1985). DSP-4 (N–(2–chloroethyl)–N–ethyl–2–bromobenzylamine) depletes noradrenaline in kitten visual cortex without altering the effects of monocular deprivation. *The Journal of Neuroscience*, **5**, 1925–33.

Daw, N. W., Robertson, T. W., Rader, R. K., Videen, T. O. & Coscia, C. J. (1984). Substantial reduction of cortical noradrenaline by lesions of adrenergic pathway does not prevent effects of monocular deprivation. *The Journal of Neuroscience*, **4**, 1354–60.

Daw, N. W., Videen, T. O., Robertson, T. & Rader, R. K. (1985a). An evaluation of the hypothesis that noradrenaline affects plasticity in the developing visual cortex. In *The Visual System* (pp. 133–44). New York: Liss.

Daw, N. W., Videen, T. O., Rader, R. K., Robertson, T. W. & Coscia, C. J. (1985b). Subtantial reduction of noradrenaline in kitten visual cortex by intraventricular injections of 6–hydroxydopamine does not always prevent ocular dominance shifts after monocular deprivation. *Experimental Brain Research*, **59**, 30–5.

Dehay, C., Horsburgh, G., Berland, M., Killackey, H. P. & Kennedy, H. (1989). Maturation and connectivity of the visual cortex in monkey is altered by prenatal removal of retinal input. *Nature, London*, **337**, 265–7.

Dehay, C., Kennedy, H. & Bullier, J. (1986). Callosal connectivity of areas V1 and V2 in the newborn monkey. *Journal of Comparative Neurology*, **254**, 20–33.

Dehay, C., Kennedy, H., Bullier, J. & Berland, M. (1988). Absence of interhemispheric connections of area 17 during development in the monkey. *Nature, London*, **331**, 348–50.

Dews, P. B. & Wiesel, T. M. (1970). Consequences of monocular deprivation on visual behavior in kittens. *Journal of Physiology*, **206**, 437–55.

Dykes, R. W., Landry, P., Metherate, R. & Hicks, T. P. (1984). Functional role of GABA in cat primary somatosensory cortex: Shaping receptive fields of cortical neurons. *Journal of Neurophysiology*, **52**, 1066–93.

Floeter, M. K. & Jones, E. G. (1985). Transplantation of fetal postmitotic neurons to rat cortex: Survival, early pathways choices and long-term projections of outgrowing axons. *Developmental Brain Research*, **22**, 19–38.

Freeman, R. D. & Bonds, A. B. (1979). Cortical plasticity in monocularly deprived immobilized kittens depends on eye movement. *Science*, **206**, 1093–5.

Glickstein, M. & Whitteridge, D. (1976). Degeneration of layer III pyramidal cells in area 18 following destruction of callosal input. *Brain Research*, **104**, 148–51.

Gorgels, T. G. M. F., De Kort, E. J. M., Van Aanholt, H. T. H. & Nieuwenhuys, R. (1989). A quantitative analysis of the development of the pyramidal tract in the cervical spinal cord in the rat. *Anatomy and Embryology*, **179**, 377–85.

Guillery, R. W. & Kaas, J. H. (1971). A study of normal and congenitally abnormal retinogeniculate projections in cats. *Journal of Comparative Neurology*, **143**, 73–100.

Hendry, S. H. C. & Jones, E. G. (1986). Reduction in number of immunostained GABAergic neurones in deprived-eye dominance columns of monkey area 17. *Nature, London*, **320**, 750–3.

(1988). Activity-dependent regulation of GABA expression in the visual cortex of adult monkeys. *Neuron*, **1**, 701–12.

Hendry, S. H. C., Jones, E. G., Killackey, H. P. & Chalupa, L. M. (1987*a*). Choline acetyl transferase immunoreactive neurons in fetal monkey cerebral cortex. *Developmental Brain Research*, **37**, 313–17.

Hendry, S. H. C., Schwark, H. D., Jones, E. G. & Yan, J. (1987*b*). Numbers and proportions of GABA-immunoreactive neurons in different areas of monkey cerebral cortex. *The Journal of Neuroscience*, **7**, 1503–19.

Horton, J. C. & Hedley-Whyte, E. T. (1984). Mapping of cytochrome oxidase patches and ocular dominance columns in human visual cortex. *Philosophical Transactions of the Royal Society, London Biology*, **304**, 255–72.

Hubel, D. H. & Wiesel, T. N. (1977). Functional architecture of macaque monkey visual cortex. *Proceedings of the The Royal Society of London (Biology)*, **198**, 1–59.

Hubel, D. H., Wiesel, T. N. & LeVay, S. (1977). Plasticity of ocular dominance columns in monkey striate cortex, *Philosophical Transactions of The Royal Society, London, Biology*, **278**, 131–63.

Huntley, G. W., Hendry, S. H. C., Killackey, H. P., Chalupa, L. M. & Jones, E. G. (1988*a*). Temporal sequence of neurotransmitter expression by developing neurons of fetal monkey visual cortex. *Developmental Brain Research*, **43**, 69–96.

(1988*b*). GABA, neuropeptide, and tyrosine hydroxylase immunoreactivity in the frontal cortex of fetal monkeys. *Neuroscience Abstracts*, **14**, 1021.

Huntley, G. W., Jones, E. G. & DeBlas, A. I. (1990). GABA receptor immunoreactivity in adult and developing monkey sensory-motor cortex. *Experimental Brain Research*, **82**, 519–35.

Innocenti, G. M. (1981). Growth and reshaping of axons in the establishment of callosal connections. *Science*, **212**, 824–7.

Innocenti, G. M. & Caminiti, R. (1980). Postnatal shaping of callosal connections from sensory areas. *Experimental Brain Research*, **38**, 381–94.

Innocenti, G. M. & Clarke, S. (1984). Bilateral transitory projection to visual areas from auditory cortex in kittens. *Developmental Brain Research*, **14**, 143–8.

Innocenti, G. M., Clarke, S. & Kraftsik, R. (1986). Interchange of callosal and association projections in the developing visual cortex. *The Journal of Neuroscience*, **6**, 1384–409.

Innocenti, G. M. & Frost, D. O. (1979). Effects of visual experience on the maturation of the efferent system to the corpus callosum. *Nature, London*, **280**, 231–3.

Jones, E. G., Valentino, K. L. & Fleshman, J. W. (1982). Adjustment of connectivity in rat neocortex after prenatal destruction of precursor cells of layers II-IV. *Developmental Brain Research*, **2**, 425–31.

Kasamatsu, T., Pettigrew, J. D. & Ary, M. (1979). Restoration of visual cortical plasticity by local microperfusion of norepinephrine. *Journal of Comparative Neurology*, **185**, 163–82.

Kass, J. H., Merzenich, M. M. & Killackey, H. P. (1983). The reorganization of the somatosensory cortex following peripheral nerve damage in adult and developing mammals. *Annual Review of Neuroscience*, **6**, 325–56.

Kelahan, A. M. & Doetsch, G. S. (1984). Time-dependent changes in the functional organization of somatosensory cerebral cortex following digit amputation in adult raccoons. *Somatosensory Research*, **2**, 49–81.

Killackey, H. P. & Chalupa, L. M. (1986). Ontogenetic change in the distribution of callosal projection neurons in the postcentral gyrus of the fetal rhesus monkey. *Journal of Comparative Neurology*, **244**, 331–48.

Killackey, H., Ivy, G. O. & Cunningham, T. J. (1978). Anomalous organization of SMI somatotopic map consequent to vibrissae removal in the newborn rat. *Brain Research*, **155**, 136–40.

Kristt, D. A. & Molliver, M. E. (1976). Synapses in newborn rat cerebral cortex: a quantitative ultrastructural study. *Brain Research*, **108**, 180–6.

LeVay, S., Wiesel, T. N. & Hubel, D. H. (1980). The development of ocular dominance columns in normal and visually deprived monkeys. *Journal of Comparative Neurology*, **191**, 1–51.

Lipton, S. A. & Kater, S. B. (1989). Neurotransmitter regulation of neuronal outgrowth, plasticity and survival, *Trends in Neuroscience*, **12(7)**, 265–9.

Lund, R. D. & Mustari, M. J. (1977). Development of the genoculocortical pathway in rats. *Journal of Comparative Neurology*, **173**, 289–306.

Lund, R. D., Mitchell, D. E. & Henry, G. H. (1978). Squint-induced modification of callosal connections in cats. *Brain Research*, **144**, 169–72.

Luskin, M. B., Pearlman, A. L. & Sanes, J. R. (1988). Cell lineage in the cerebral cortex of the mouse studied *in vivo* and *in vitro* with a recombinant retrovirus. *Neuron*, **1**, 635–47.

Marin-Padilla, M. (1984). Neurons of layer I. A developmental analysis. In: A. Peters & E. G. Jones (Eds.), *Cerebral Cortex, Volume I: Cellular Components of the Cerebral Cortex* (pp. 447–78). New York: Plenum.

(1988). Early ontogenesis of the human cerebral cortex. In: A. Peters & E. G. Jones (Eds.), *Cerebral Cortex, Volume 7: Development and Maturation of Cerebral Cortex* (pp. 1–34). New York: Plenum.

McConnell, S. K. (1985). Migration and differentiation of cerebral cortical neurons after transplantation into the brains of ferrets. *Science*, **229**, 1268–71.

(1988). Fates of visual cortical neurons in the ferret after isochronic and heterochronic transplantation. *The Journal of Neuroscience*, **8**, 945–74.

McConnell, S. K., Ghosh, A. & Shatz, C. J. (1989). Subplate neurons pioneer the first axon pathway from the cerebral cortex. *Science* **245**, 978–81.

McKinley, P. A. & Kruger, L. (1988). Nonoverlapping thalamocortical connections to normal and deprived primary somatosensory cortex for similar forelimb receptive fields in chronic spinal cats. *Somatosensory Research*, **5**, 311–23.

Merzenich, M. M., Kaas, J. H., Wall, J., Nelson, R. J., Sur, M. & Felleman, D. (1983*a*). Topographic reorganization of somatosensory cortical areas 3B and 1 in adult monkeys following restricted deafferentiation. *Neuroscience*, **8**, 33–56.

Merzenich, M. M., Kaas, J. H., Wall, J. T., Sur, M., Nelson, R. J. & Felleman, D. J. (1983*b*). Progression of change following median nerve section in the cortical representation of the hand in areas 3b and 1 in adult owl and squirrel monkeys. *Neuroscience*, **10**, 639–66.

Merzenich, M. M., Nelson, R. J., Stryker, M. P., Cynader, M. S., Schoppmann, A. & Zook, J. M. (1984). Somatosensory cortical map changes following digit amputation in adult monkeys. *Journal of Comparative Neurology*, **224**, 591–605.

Merzenich, M. M., Recanzone, G., Jenkins, W. M., Allard, T. & Nudo, R. J. (1988). Cortical representational plasticity. In J. P. Changeux and M. Konishi, eds., *The Neural and Molecular Basis for Learning*. Chichester, England: John Wiley and Sons.

Mountcastle, V. B. (1978). An organizing principle for cerebral function: The unit module and the distributed system. In G. M. Edelman and V. B. Mountcastle, *The Mindful Brain. Cortical Organization and the Group-Selective Theory of Higher Brain Function*, pp. 7–50. Cambridge, MA: MIT Press.

Movshon, J. A. and van Sluyters, R. C. (1981). Visual neuronal development, *Annual Review of Psychology*, **32**, 477–522.

O'Kusky, J. & Colonnier, M. (1982*a*). A laminar analysis of the number of neurons, glia, and synapses in the visual cortex (area 17) of adult macaque monkeys. *Journal of Comparative Neurology*, **210**, 278–90.

(1982*b*). Postnatal changes in the number of neurons and synapses in the visual cortex (Area 17) of the macaque monkey: A stereological analysis in normal and monocularly deprived animals. *Journal of Comparative Neurology*, **210**, 291–505.

Olavarria, J. & van Sluyters, R. (1985). Organization and postnatal development of callosal connections in the visual cortex of the rat. *Journal of Comparative Neurology*, **239**, 1–26.

O'Leary, D. D. M. & Stanfield, B. B. (1985). Occipital cortical neurons with transient pyramidal tract axons extend and maintain collaterals to subcortical but not intracortical targets. *Brain Research*, **336**, 326–33.

(1986). A transient pyramidal tract projection from the visual cortex in the hamster and its removal by selective collateral elimination. *Developmental Brain Research*, **27**, 87–100.

O'Leary, D. D. M., Stanfield, B. B. & Cowan, W. M. (1981). Evidence that the early postnatal restriction of the cells of origin of the callosal projection is due to the elimination of axonal collaterals rather than to the death of neurons. *Developmental Brain Research*, **1**, 607–17.

Price, J. & Thurlow, L. (1988). Cell lineage in the rat cerebral cortex: A study using retroviral-mediated gene transfer. *Development*, **104**, 473–82.

Rakic, P. (1972). Mode of cell migration to the superficial layers of fetal monkey neocortex. *Journal of Comparative Neurology*, **145**, 61–84.

(1974). Neurons in rhesus monkey visual cortex: systematic relation between time of origin and eventual disposition. *Science*, **183**, 425–7.

(1981). Development of visual centers in the primate brain depends on binocular competition before birth. *Science*, **214**, 928–31.

(1988). Specification of cerebral cortical areas. *Science*, **241**, 170–6.

Rakic, P. & Goldman-Rakic, P. S. (1982). Development and modifiability of the cerebral cortex. *Neuroscience Research Progress Bulletin*, **20**, 433–606.

Rakic, P., Bourgeois, J.-P., Eckenhoff, M. F., Zecevic, N. & Goldman-Rakic, P. S. (1986). Concurrent overproduction of synapses in diverse regions of the primate cerebral cortex. *Science*, **231**, 232–5.

Rauschecker, J. P. & Singer, W. (1982). The effects of early visual experience on the cat's visual cortex and their possible explanation by Hebb synapses. *Journal of Physiology (London)*, **310**, 215–39.

Reh, T. & Kalil, K. (1981). Development of the pyramidal tract in the hamster: I. A light microscopic study. *Journal of Comparative Neurology*, **200**, 55–67.

(1982). Development of the pyramidal tract in the hamster: II. An electron microscopic study. *Journal of Comparative Neurology*, **205**, 77–88.

Rockel, A. J., Hiorns, R. W. & Powell, T. P. S. (1974). Numbers of neurons through full depth of neocortex. *Journal of Anatomy*, **118**, 371.

(1980). The basic uniformity in structure of the neocortex. *Brain*, **103**, 221–44.

Schlumpf, M., Shoemaker, W. J. & Bloom, F. E. (1980). Innervation of embryonic rat cerebral cortex by catecholamine-containing fibers. *Journal of Comparative Neurology*, **192**, 361–76.

Schreyer, D. J. & Jones, E. G. (1982). Growth and target finding by axons of the corticospinal tract in the prenatal and postnatal rat. *Neuroscience*, **7**, 1837–53.

(1988a). Axon elimination in the developing corticospinal tract of the rat. *Development Brain Research*, **38**, 103–19.

(1988b). Topographic sequence of outgrowth of corticospinal axons in the rat: A study using retrograde axonal labeling with Fast Blue. *Developmental Brain Research*, **38**, 89–101.

Schwartz, M. L. & Goldman-Rakic, P. S. (1988). Some callosal neurons of the fetal monkey frontal cortex have axons in the contralateral hemisphere prior to the completion of migration. *Neuroscience Abstracts*, **12**, 1211.

Schwartz, M. L., Zheng, D.-S. & Goldman-Rakic, P. S. (1988). Periodicity of GABA-containing cells in primate prefrontal cortex. *Journal of Neuroscience*, **8**, 1962–70.

Shatz, C. (1977a). A comparison of visual pathways in Boston and midwestern Siamese cats. *Journal of Comparative Neurology*, **171**, 205–28.

(1977b). Abnormal interhemispheric connections in the visual system of

Boston Siamese cats: a physiological study. *Journal of Comparative Neurology*, **171**, 229–46.

Shatz, C. J. & Luskin, M. B. (1986). The relationship between the geniculocortical afferents and their cortical target cells during development of the cat's primary visual cortex. *The Journal of Neuroscience*, **6**, 3655–68.

Shaw, C., Needler, M. D. & Cynader, M. (1984). Ontogenesis of muscimol binding sites in cat visual cortex. *Brain Research Bulletin*, **13**, 331–4.

Shaw, C., Wilkinson, M., Cynader, M., Needler, M. C., Aoki, C. & Hall, S. E. (1986). The laminar distributions and postnatal development of neurotransmitter and neuromodulator receptors in cat visual cortex, *Brain Research Bulletin*, **16**, 661–71.

Sherman, S. M. & Spear, P. D. (1982). Organization of visual pathways in normal and visual deprived cats. *Physiological Review*, **62**, 738–855.

Shoumura, K. (1974). An attempt to relate the origin and distribution of commissural fibers to the presence of large and medium pyramids in layer III in the cat's visual cortex. *Brain Research*, **67**, 13–25.

Shoumura, K., Ando, T. & Kato, K. (1975). Structural organization of 'callosal' OBg in human corpus callosum agenesis. *Brain Research*, **93**, 241–52.

Sillito, A. M. (1975). The contribution of inhibitory mechanisms to the receptive field properties of neurones in the striate cortex of the cat. *Journal of Physiology (London)*, **250**, 305–29.

(1979). Inhibitory mechanisms influencing complex cell orientation selectivity and their modification at high resting discharge levels. *Journal of Physiology (London)*, **289**, 33–53.

Sillito, A. M., Kemp, J. A. & Blakemore, C. (1981). The role of GABAergic inhibition in the cortical effects of monocular deprivation. *Nature, London*, **291**, 318–20.

Singer, W. (1988). Pattern recognition and self-organization in biological systems. H. Marks *et al.* (Eds.), *Processing Structures for Perception and Action.* (pp. 1–18). Weinheim: VCH.

Snow, P. J., Nudo, R. J., Rivers, W., Jenkins, W. M. & Merzenich, M. M. (1988). Somatotopically inappropriate projections from thalamocortical neurons to SI cortex of the cat demonstrated by the use of intracortical microstimulation. *Somatosensory Research*, **5**, 349–72.

Stanfield, B. B., O'Leary, D. D. M. & Fricks, C. (1982). Selective collateral elimination in early postnatal development restricts cortical distribution of rat pyramidal tract neurones. *Nature, London*, **298**, 371–3.

Stryker, M. P. & Harris, W. A. (1986). Binocular impulse blockade prevents the formation of ocular dominance columns in cat visual cortex. *The Journal of Neuroscience*, **6**, 2117.

Stryker, M. P. & Strickland, S. L. (1984). Physiological segregation of ocular dominance columns depends on the pattern of afferent electrical activity. *Investigations in Ophthalmology Supplement*, **25**, 278.

Van der Loos, H. & Woolsey, T. A. (1973). Somatosensory cortex: structural alterations following early injury to sense organs. *Science*, **179**, 395–8.

Verney, C., Berger, B., Adrien, J., Vigny, A. & Gay, M. (1982). Development of the dopaminergic innervation of the rat cerebral cortex. A light microscopic immunocytochemical study using anti-tyrosine hydroxylase antibodies. *Developmental Brain Research*, **5**, 41–52.

Videen, T. O., Daw, N. W. & Rader, R. K. (1984). The effect of norepinephrine on visual cortical neurons in kittens and adult cats. *The Journal of Neuroscience*, **4**, 1607–17.

Walsh, C. & Cepko, C. L. (1988). Clonally related cortical cells show several migration patterns, *Science*, **241**, 1342–5.

Wiesel, T. N. & Hubel, D. H. (1965). Comparison of the effects of unilateral and bilateral closure on cortical unit responses in kittens. *Journal of Neurophysiology*, **28**, 1029–40.

Winfield, D. A. (1981). The postnatal development of synapses in the visual cortex of cats and the effects of eyelid closure, *Brain Research*, **206**, 349–52.

Wise, S. P., Hendry, S. H. C. & Jones, E. G. (1977). Prenatal development of sensorimotor cortical projections in cats. *Brain Research*, **138**, 538–44.

Wise, S. P. & Jones, E. G. (1976). The organization and postnatal development of the commissural projection of the rat somatic sensory cortex. *Journal of Comparative Neurology*, **163**, 313–44.

    (1978). Developmental studies of thalamocortical and commissural connections in the rat somatic sensory cortex. *Journal of Comparative Neurology*, **178**, 187–208.

Yurkewicz, L., Valentino, K. L., Floeter, M. K., Fleshman, J. W., Jr. & Jones, E. G. (1984). Effects of cytotoxic deletions of somatic sensory cortex in fetal rats. *Somatosensory Research*, **1**, 303–27.

Part III

Genetic and teratogenic disturbances in fetal neural development

4

Genetic disturbances of neuronal migration: some examples from the limbic system of mutant mice

RICHARD S. NOWAKOWSKI

Robert Wood Johnson Medical School

Introduction

Single gene mutations in the mouse affect the development of the CNS in a variety of ways. For most available mouse mutants, the gene action in the developing CNS produces an adult brain which is functionally compromised. In fact, most neurological mutations in the mouse produce *overt* changes in the behavior of the animal, mostly involving locomotory behavior. The reason for this is quite simply that these obvious behavioral changes are most easily detected and/or screened for in large mouse colonies. For example, there are many mouse mutants known that affect the development of the cerebellar cortex (e.g. Caviness & Rakic, 1978; Herrup, 1983; Mullen & Herrup, 1979). In fact, the availability of this variety of mutations is one of the major reasons that so much is known about cerebellar development. Similarly large collections of available mouse mutants are known that affect the development of the vestibular system and other areas and which produce problems in locomotion (M. C. Green, 1981).

Unfortunately, a comparably extensive assortment of mutations that affect the development of the cerebral cortex has not been available. Indeed, until recently only the reeler mutation (gene symbol: *rl*) was known to affect the development of the cerebral cortex (Caviness & Sidman, 1973*a*, and *b*; Caviness & Rakic, 1978; Pearlman, 1985). In the case of reeler, the mutation is an autosomal recessive gene that affects neuronal migration in many parts of the CNS (Caviness, 1973, 1982, 1986; Stanfield & Cowan, 1979*a* and *b*; Stanfield, Caviness & Cowan, 1979). The main reason that there are so few mutations known to affect the development of the cerebral cortex is the fact

69

that apparently such mutations generally produce only *covert* behavioral changes, i.e. changes that are not easily detectable upon routine observation of the animal. Reeler is a notable exception in that *rl/rl* mice display obvious motor deficits.

Recently, however, several new genetically-based disturbances of cerebral cortical development have been described (Nowakowski, 1988). These new mutations have been discovered by comparing the anatomy of the hippocampus in inbred strains of mice. These comparisons provide a standard against which to judge what is normal and what is abnormal, and have resulted in the identification of new mutations which affect cell proliferation and cell migration. Each of these mutations is being analyzed to answer a variety of developmental questions. This review will concentrate on understanding how the abnormally-positioned cells resulting from disruptions of neuronal migration make and receive connections with their normally-positioned targets in other parts of the brain.

What is an inbred strain?

Inbred strains of mice were first produced in the early part of the twentieth century as a way to study the genetic basis for cancer and for the variety of coat colors that exist in wild-type mice (Staats, 1966). The typical method used to create an inbred strain is illustrated in Fig. 4.1. Essentially this involves choosing two parent mice from a wild population and then brother–sister mating their progeny for twenty consecutive generations. With each successive generation two things happen: (1) the amount of genetic diversity among the offspring is reduced, and (2) various genes which exist in heterozygous forms in the wild-type mouse are forced to homozygosity in the inbred offspring. After twenty generations of brother–sister mating, two siblings are alike at 98% of their genetic loci, and each inbred mouse has 99.9% of its genes forced to homozygosity (E. Green, 1981). During the process of inbreeding, however, the genes which are forced to homozygosity differ in each of the inbred strains that are made (Fig. 4.1). Thus, each inbred strain has a different subset of alleles at each of the various genetic loci, but within each inbred strain the siblings are essentially genetically identical. Since the turn of the century, several hundred inbred strains have been made (M. C. Green, 1981), and each strain can be considered to carry a sample of the genes that are present in a normal wild population of mice. The more common inbred strains (e.g. C57BL/6J and BALB/cJ) have been inbred for well over 100 generations.

Because the animals of an inbred strain provide an opportunity to make a large number of observations on essentially genetically identical individuals,

What is an inbred strain?

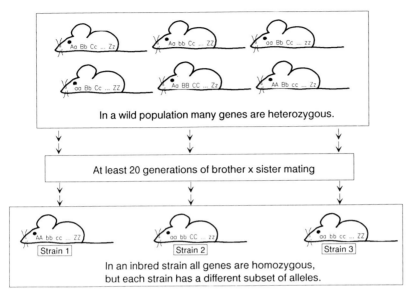

In a wild population many genes are heterozygous.

At least 20 generations of brother x sister mating

Strain 1   Strain 2   Strain 3

In an inbred strain all genes are homozygous,
but each strain has a different subset of alleles.

Figure 4.1. General strategy for producing an inbred strain of mice. (For further details, see text.)

the 'normal' anatomy, development, physiology, etc., of any particular structure can be defined as that exhibited by virtually all animals of a particular inbred strain. In the case of the anatomy and development of the hippocampal formation, normal has been defined arbitrarily as the hippocampal formation of a mouse of the C57BL/6J inbred strain. There is, of course, no *a priori* reason for contending that the brains of C57BL/6J mice are 'more normal' than those of any other inbred strain. However, the Jackson Laboratory (Bar Harbor, Me.) maintains many mutants on this strain, which is one of the most widely-available of the inbred strains. Also, an excellent atlas of the CNS of the C57BL/6J mouse is available (Sidman, Angevine & Taber-Pierce, 1971). C57BL/6J is, therefore, a convenient standard, and as such has become, *de facto*, the normal mouse for neurological analysis.

The normal hippocampal formation

Anatomy

The hippocampal formation of a C57BL/6J mouse in horizontal section is illustrated in Fig. 4.2. In horizontal sections, about two-thirds of the hippocampal formation of the brain of a laboratory rodent is cut orthogonal to its major axis, as defined by Lorente de No (1934); thus the horizontal plane is the most appropriate for studies of this structure. The major subdivisions of the hippocampal formation are the dentate gyrus, the hippocampus, and the subiculum (Angevine, 1965). The main cellular layer of the dentate gyrus is the horseshoe-shaped granule cell layer. External to the granule cell layer is the molecular layer, and internal to it is the hilus (or area CA4). The hippocampus is subdivided into areas CA1, CA2 and CA3. From ventricle to pia, the laminae of the hippocampus are: the alveus; the stratum oriens; the pyramidal cell layer; the stratum radiatum; and the stratum lacunosum-moleculare. In area CA3 there is an additional lamina, the stratum lucidum, which is situated between the pyramidal cell layer and the stratum radiatum and which contains the mossy fibers arising from the granule cells of the dentate gyrus. This highly laminated organization of the hippocampal formation of the normal mouse makes it an ideal location in which to assess the affects of mutant genes on the process of cell migration during the development of the CNS.

Development

The normal development of the hippocampal formation has been studied extensively in a variety of species (Cowan, Stanfield & Kishi, 1980; Rickmann, Amaral & Cowan, 1987; Nowakowski & Rakic, 1981; Nowakowski, 1988; Bayer, 1980a,b). As in all other regions of the CNS, the developmental process entails three basic cellular mechanisms: (1) cell

Figure 4.2. A. Horizontal section through the hippocampal formation of an adult C57BL/6J mouse. B. Schematic diagram illustrating the major subdivisions and laminae of the hippocampal formation. The borders between subdivisions are indicated in both A and B by arrows. Abbreviations: F, fimbria; GCL, granule cell layer; HF, hippocampal fissure; LV, lateral ventricle; ML, molecular layer; NCx, neocortex; PCL, pyramidal cell layer; PRE, presubiculum; SL, stratum lucidum; SO, stratum oriens; SR, stratum radiatum; SUB, subiculum; THAL, thalamus. (Reproduced from Nowakowski, 1988.)

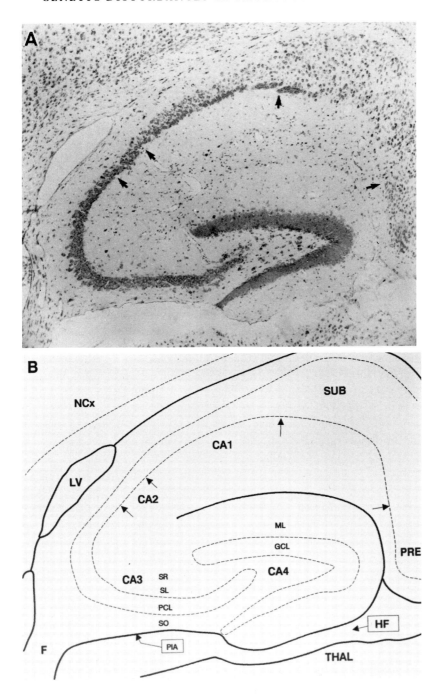

proliferation; (2) cell migration; and (3) cell differentiation (see Chapter 2). Except for the granule cells of the dentate gyrus, the neurons of the hippocampal formation are generated during characteristic prenatal intervals in the mouse (Angevine, 1965; Nowakowski, 1985; see Fig. 4.3, top) as well as in other species (Rakic & Nowakowski, 1981; Bayer, 1980a,b; Schlessinger, Cowan & Gottlieb, 1975; Wyss & Sripanidkulchai, 1985). Most of the dentate gyrus granule cells are generated postnatally during the first 30 days after birth (Angevine, 1965), although there is evidence in the rat that this period may be considerably longer (Kaplan & Hinds, 1977; Bayer, Yackel & Puri, 1982). All of the neurons of the hippocampal formation are generated in one of two proliferative zones (see Nowakowski, this volume). Most of the neurons, including all of the hippocampal pyramidal cells, are generated in the ventricular zone lining the lateral ventricle (Nowakowski & Rakic, 1981; Rakic & Nowakowski, 1981). In contrast, while some of the granule cells of the dentate gyrus are generated in the ventricular zone, most are generated in an intrahilar proliferative zone (Nowakowski & Rakic, 1981; Eckenhoff & Rakic, 1984). It is important to note, however, that the proliferating cells that comprise the intrahilar proliferative zone are themselves derived from the ventricular zone (Nowakowski & Rakic, 1981).

In order to reach either the intrahilar proliferative zone or their final adult positions, the neuroblasts and young neurons produced in the ventricular zone migrate along radial glial fibers across a complicated terrain (Nowakowski & Rakic, 1979; Rickmann et al., 1987). The migratory pathways followed by neurons destined to reside in the subiculum and areas CA1 and CA2 are fairly direct (Nowakowski, 1985). The migratory path followed by neurons that are destined to reside in area CA3, however, not only is tortuous but lengthens even as the young neurons move along it to their ultimate destination (Fig. 4.3, bottom; see Nowakowski, 1985; Rickmann et al., 1987). The young neurons destined for the dentate gyrus and the neuroblasts destined for the intrahilar proliferative zone pursue a migratory path which is adjacent to the pathway followed by the CA3-bound neurons but situated closer to the pial surface of the transverse fissure. Thus, while the cells destined for area CA3 and the dentate gyrus migrate along radially-oriented glial fibers, their movement is along a path which is initially perpendicular to the ventricular surface but which is largely parallel to a pial surface because of the distortions produced by the growing hippocampus and dentate gyrus. In other words, the topographic representation of the subdivisions of the adult hippocampal formation is reflected in an orientation perpendicular to the pial surface of the hippocampal fissure in the organization of the radial glial cells and their apposed migrating neurons. This relationship between a topographic representation and the pial surface is unique in the cerebral cortex.

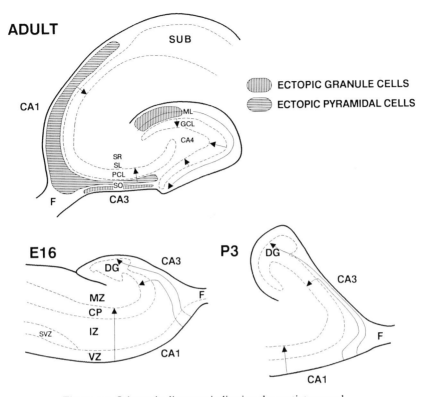

Figure 4.3. Schematic diagrams indicating the spatiotemporal gradients and migratory pathways of neurons comprising the mouse hippocampal formation. In the drawing at the top, the arrows indicate in the adult the direction of the spatiotemporal gradient of neuron origin; the tip of the arrowhead indicates the position of the last-born neurons, while the tail of the arrow indicates the position of the first-born neurons. Shaded areas indicate the cytoarchitectonic positions in which ectopic neurons are found in a variety of mouse mutants. (For details, see text.) In the bottom two drawings, arrows illustrate the migratory pathways from the ventricular zone (VZ) to areas CA1, CA3, and the dentate gyrus (DG) followed by young neurons on E16 and P3 (Nowakowski, 1988). Abbreviations: CP, cortical plate; F, fimbria; GCL, granule cell layer; IZ, intermediate zone; ML, molecular layer; MZ, marginal zone; PCL, pyramidal cell layer; SL, stratum lucidum; SO, stratum oriens; SR, stratum radiatum; SUB, subiculum; SVZ, subventricular zone; VZ, ventricular zone.

75

Table 4.1. *Eight murine migration mutants that are known to affect neuronal migration in the developing hippocampal formation.*

Gene symbol	Gene name	Chromosome	Genetic background
dr^{sst-J}	dreher	1	C3B6/J(N17)
Hld	Hippocampal lamination defect	—	BALB/cByJ
rl^{ORL}	reeler	5	Noninbred
—	—	—	NZB/BlNJ
bal	balding	—	C57BL/6J
Lps^d	Lipopolysaccharide response defect	4	C3H/HeJ
me^v	viable motheaten	6	C57BL/6J
bg	beige	13	C57BL/6J

Hippocampal mutants

The development of the hippocampal formation is known to be affected by seven mutations and one genetic variant (see Table 4.1), all of which share the phenotypic characteristic of neuronal ectopia. The presence of ectopic neurons indicates that the process of neuronal migration is disrupted either directly or indirectly by each of these mutations.

The Hippocampal lamination defect mutation

Of the mutations known to affect neuronal migration, the Hippocampal lamination defect mutation (gene symbol: *Hld*) produces the most localized effect on the development of the hippocampal formation. This autosomal dominant mutation (Nowakowski, 1984) is characterized by an inversion of the laminar organization of the pyramidal cell layer of area CA3c. This inversion is the result of a disruption of migration of only those late-generated pyramidal cells destined for area CA3c (Fig. 4.4); the late-generated pyramidal cells destined for area CA1, as well as all of the early-generated cells, are normally positioned (Barber *et al.*, 1974; Vaughn *et al.*, 1977). The late-generated pyramidal cells are generated on embryonic days 15 and 16 in the proliferative zone lining the lateral ventrical in both the normal (i.e. +/+ or wild-type) and *Hld*/*Hld* mouse (Fig. 4.5). The young

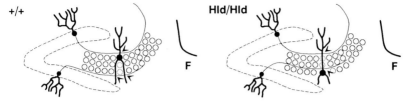

Figure 4.4. Schematic diagram indicating the position and mossy fiber input of late-generated pyramidal cells in area CA3c of wildtype ($+/+$) and Hld/Hld mutant mice. In $+/+$ mice (left), late-generated pyramidal cells occupy the top of the pyramidal cell layer and receive mossy fiber input at two positions (arrowheads): on their apical dendrites, where they pass through the suprapyramidal mossy fiber layer; and on their basal dendrites, where they pass through the infrapyramidal mossy fiber layer. In Hld/Hld mice (right) late-generated pyramidal cells fail to migrate past earlier generated ones and occupy the bottom of the pyramidal cell layer in area CA3c. These ectopic pyramidal cells receive mossy fiber input at two positions on their apical dendrites (arrowheads), once where they pass through the suprapyramidal mossy fiber layer and once where they pass through the infrapyramidal mossy fiber layer (Source: Nowakowski, 1988; Nowakowski & Davis, 1985).

neurons destined for area CA3c leave the ventricular zone and migrate across a broad intermediate zone until they reach the border with the developing cortical plate after approximately seven days (Nowakowski, 1985). In the $+/+$ mouse they continue to migrate past the previously generated pyramidal cells to take up their final position at the top of the cortical plate; in the Hld/Hld mouse, however, they stop migrating, do not bypass the previously generated cells, and remain in a position *below* the early-generated pyramidal cells. Thus, the ectopic pyramidal cells of area CA3c migrate along their normal migratory pathway and at a normal speed but stop prematurely (Nowakowski, 1985).

The dreher mutant mouse

A markedly different reorganization of hippocampal anatomy is seen in the dreher mutation (gene symbol: dr). This autosomal recessive gene produces considerable variation in phenotype even among genetically identical mice in both homozygotes (Wahlsten, Lyons & Zagaja, 1983) and heterozygotes (Patrylo, Sekiguchi & Nowakowski, 1990). In dr/dr mice both cell proliferation and neuronal migration of the granule cells of the dentate gyrus and the pyramidal cells of the hippocampus are affected. In the dentate gyrus, large

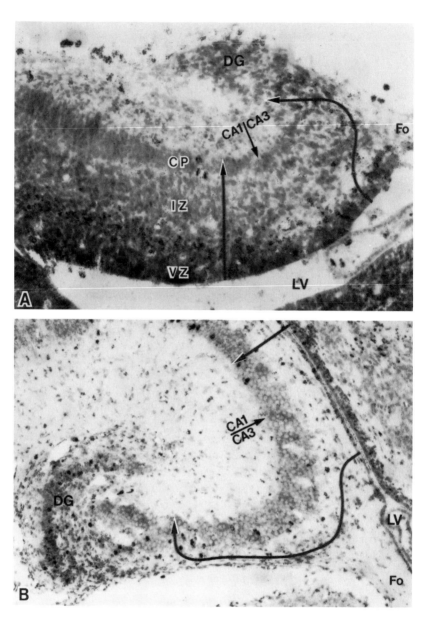

Figure 4.5. Photomicrographs of the hippocampal formation of the mouse at E16 (A) and P3 (B). In each micrograph the arrows extend from the ventricular zone to the top of the cortical plate and indicate the migratory path followed by neurons at that age to areas CA3c and CA1. Late-generated neurons begin their migration at E16 and are close to completing that migration at P3. Note that during this period the length of the migratory path to area CA3c increases considerably while the length of the migratory path to area CA1 remains approximately the same, or perhaps decreases slightly. Abbreviations: CP, cortical plate; Fo, fornix; IZ, intermediate zone; LV, lateral ventricle; VZ, ventricular zone (Nowakowski, 1985).

78

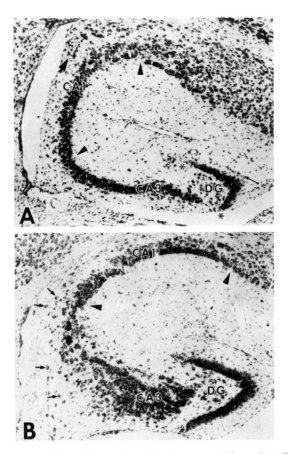

Figure 4.6. Photomicrographs of the hippocampal formation of dreher mutant mice illustrate the morphological variation seen among *dr/dr* mice. A. In this specimen parts of the both the suprapyramidal and infrapyramidal granule cell layers of the dentate gyrus (DG) are missing (asterisks), there are ectopic granule cells in the molecular layer of the dentate gyrus (thin arrow), and there are ectopic pyramidal cells in the stratum oriens underlying area CA1 (heavy arrow). B. In this specimen there are numerous ectopic pyramidal cells in the stratum oriens underlying area CA3 (arrows), and the pyramidal cell layer of area CA3 is abnormally thick. (Modified from Nowakowski, 1988.)

portions of the granule cell layer are often missing, and there are often small clusters of granule cells abnormally positioned in the molecular layer (Fig. 4.6A, B). Most frequently the infrapyramidal limb of the dentate gyrus is absent; when this happens it is apparent in Timm's-stained preparations that the infrapyramidal mossy fiber layer also is absent (Nowakowski & Wahlsten, 1985a,b). In area CA3 there are sometimes too few neurons and sometimes too many. When there are too many pyramidal cells, there are often pyramidal neurons and sometimes even granule cells abnormally positioned in the stratum oriens (Fig. 4.6B). These abnormally-positioned cells seem to be distributed along their normal migratory pathways. Interestingly, Timm's-stained preparations indicate that the abnormally-positioned granule cells send a small bundle of mossy fibers to terminate on the abnormally-positioned pyramidal cells (Nowakowski & Wahlsten, 1985a,b). Curiously, they do not seem to send any input to the basal dendrites of normally-positioned CA3c pyramidal neurons even though this otherwise normal target is closer. Experiments using tritiated thymidine autoradiography to elucidate the nature of the developmental abnormality in dreher have demonstrated that: (1) the abnormally-positioned pyramidal cells in the stratum oriens are late-generated; and (2) within the pyramidal cell layer of area CA3, the late-generated pyramidal neurons fail to bypass the early-generated ones (Nowakowski, unpublished observations).

Many of the CA3c pyramidal cells whose somata are situated in the pyramidal cell layer have dendritic trees which look entirely normal (Fig. 4.7, cells A and B). Such pyramidal cells have essentially normal looking apical dendrites and robust basal dendrites with dendritic excrescences similar in quantity and size to those seen in littermate controls and other normal mice. In particular, the location of the dendritic excrescences on both the basal and apical dendrites corresponds to the position of the two mossy-fiber bundles (arrows in Fig. 4.7). Some of the CA3c pyramidal cells, however, do not have normal dendritic trees (Fig. 4.7, cells C and D), even though their somata are located in the pyramidal cell layer. The most frequently observed abnormality is the occurrence of fine-caliber dendritic branches extending out of the apical dendrite (Fig. 4.7, cell D) or the apical portion of the soma (Fig. 4.7, cell C) and laterally through the pyramidal cell layer or at an upwardly directed angle towards the stratum radiatum. In addition, the basal dendrites of some cells travel laterally within the pyramidal cell layer without extensive ramification (Fig. 4.7, cell D) rather than extending into the stratum oriens and ramifying (Fig. 4.7, cell C).

The ectopic pyramidal cells in the stratum oriens usually have a single, thick, long apical dendrite. Overall, the pattern of their dendritic arbor is quite similar to that of normally-positioned pyramidal cells (Fig. 4.7, cells E and F). However, occasionally a pyramidal cell with a thin, poorly-branched

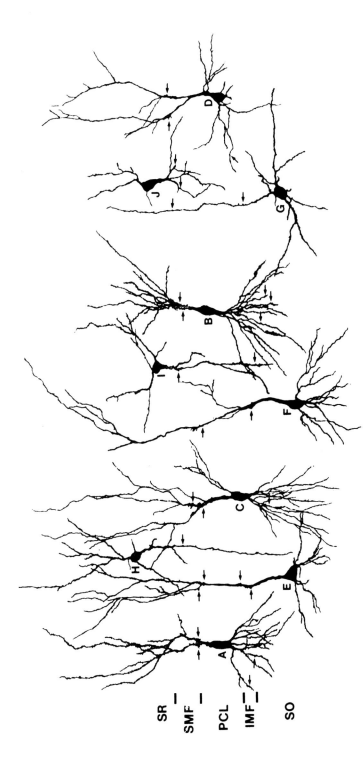

Figure 4.7. Drawings of pyramidal cells from area CA3c of a homozygous dreher (*dr/dr*) mouse. The somata of cells A through D are located within the pyramidal cell layer. The somata of cells E through G are in the stratum oriens. The somata of cells H through J are in the stratum radiatum. The arrows indicate the position of dendritic excrescences. Abbreviations: IMF, infrapyramidal mossy fiber layer; PCL, pyramidal cell layer; SMF, suprapyramidal mossy fiber layer; SO, stratum oriens; SR, stratum radiatum.

apical dendrite is seen (e.g. Fig. 4.7, cell G). Some of the cells with thick apical dendrites sometimes have fine-caliber secondary branches coming off of the apical dendrite within the pyramidal cell layer (Fig. 4.7, cell F), but others send their apical dendrites through the pyramidal cell layer without emitting such branches (Fig. 4.7, cell E).

Most of the dendritic arbors of ectopic pyramidal cells in the stratum radiatum are characterized by an inverted shape (Fig. 4.7, cells H and I). They usually have one main dendrite which extends toward the pyramidal cell layer and which bifurcates in the vicinity of the stratum lucidum (Fig. 4.7, Cells H and I). One of the branches usually extends through the pyramidal cell layer to the stratum oriens where it ends without ramifying (Fig. 4.7, cells H and I). Some of the ectopic pyramidal cells in the stratum radiatum have short, basally-directed processes which extend into but do not traverse the pyramidal cell layer (Fig. 4.7, cell J). These basally-directed dendrites frequently branch into two or three smaller branches just prior to entering the pyramidal cell layer; such cells tend to be farther from the upper border of the pyramidal cell layer.

The NZB/BlNJ inbred strain

Recently, polymorphisms indicating the existence of a mutation affecting the development of the hippocampal formation been discovered in the NZB//BlNJ inbred strain (Nowakowski, 1986, 1988). In the hippocampal formation of NZB/BlNJ mice there are abnormalities in cell position in both the dentate gyrus and the hippocampus. Clusters of abnormally-positioned granule cells are found in the molecular layer of the dentate gyrus (Fig. 4.8). These clusters of granule cells seem to be regularly spaced along the surface of the suprapyramidal limb of the dentate gyrus, although they are sometimes located along the surface of the infrapyramidal limb. In area CA3 there are small clusters of pyramidal cells abnormally positioned in the stratum lucidum and stratum radiatum (Fig. 4.8). In both the dentate gyrus and hippocampus the abnormalities in cell position occur most frequently in the ventral half of the hippocampal formation.

The existence of these abnormalities in cell position in the NZB/BlNJ inbred strain is interesting for two reasons. First, the abnormally positioned pyramidal and granule cells in NZB/BlNJ have migrated too far. This is in marked contrast to the cell position defects found in the hippocampal formation of the *Hld* and reeler mice, in which the abnormally positioned cells have not migrated far enough. Second, this abnormality in cell position in the hippocampal formation is similar to that of the neocortex of NZB/BlNJ mice, in which Sherman, Galaburda & Geschwind (1985) have described

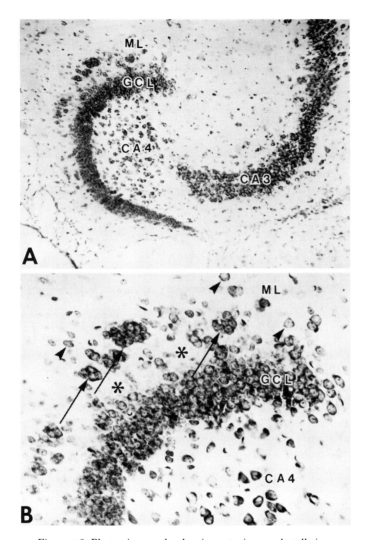

Figure 4.8. Photomicrographs showing ectopic granule cells in the molecular layer of the dentate gyrus of an NZB/B1NJ mouse. A. Low magnification of the dentate gyrus and adjacent hippocampus. Ectopic granule cells in the molecular layer are shown at higher magnification in B. While the ectopic granule cells occur mostly in clusters (arrows), they can also be found as isolated cells (arrowheads). The ectopic cells are separated from the granule cell layer by a relatively cell-sparse region of neuropil (asterisks). Abbreviations: GCL, granule cell layer; ML, molecular layer (Nowakowski, 1988).

islands of ectopic neurons in layer I of the neocortex in about 30% of NZB/BlNJ mice. Furthermore, it has been noted that there are similar ectopic clusters of neurons in the neocortex of human dyslexics, and it has been suggested that both the murine and human abnormalities may be related to autoimmune disorders (Sherman *et al.*, 1985).

We have examined the dendritic trees of the ectopic neurons in the molecular layer of the dentate gyrus of NZB/BlNJ mice and have found that they are characterized by five distinct morphological abnormalities: (1) the initial orientation of the primary dendrites can be either apical or basal; (2) the basally-directed dendrites do not reach the granule cell layer but usually curve towards the pial surface; (3) many of the dendrites end before reaching the pial surface; (4) the soma may have spines; and (5) the axon can exit from the cell body at any point or from a basal dendrite and extend up into the molecular layer. Each of the ectopic granule cells displays one or more of these abnormalities but not necessarily all of them, and the degree of expression of each type of abnormality varies from granule cell to granule cell. The dendrites that originate from the apical surface arise either as a single, main dendrite (Fig. 4.9, cell C) or as more than one process from separate areas of the cell body (Fig. 4.9, cells A, D, and E). They sometimes arborize extensively (Fig. 4.9, cell B), but usually they have only a few branches (Fig. 4.9, cells A, D, and E) which do not always reach all the way to the pial surface. Most of the ectopic granule cells have a single dendrite that extends out of the basal aspect of the ectopic neuron towards the granule cell layer (Fig. 4.9, cells A, C, D, and E). We have observed only one cell without a basal dendrite (Fig. 4.9, cell B) and no examples of an ectopic granule cell with more than one such basally-directed dendrite. In general, the basally-directed dendrite leaves the cell body from the basolateral surface that is facing the suprapyramidal tip of the granule cell layer. As a result, the basal portion of the dendritic tree is usually directed at a slight angle towards the suprapyramidal tip of the dentate gyrus. The basal dendrites are never observed to enter the granule cell layer; instead they either turn towards the pial surface (Fig. 4.9, cells A, C, and D) or run parallel to the granule cell layer (Fig. 4.9, cell E). Furthermore, the recursion of the branches back towards the pial surface almost always occurs in the same direction; they usually make their turn towards the suprapyramidal tip of the dentate gyrus (Fig. 4.9, cells A, C, and D).

The features of the dendrites of the ectopic granule cells reflect their interaction(s) with the constituents of their environment. Moreover, these interactions are similar to those documented to occur for the molecular layer interneurons of the cerebellar cortex (Rakic, 1972, 1975). For example, the orientation of the apical and basal dendrites of the ectopic granule cells with respect to the suprapyramidal-to-infrapyramidal spatiotemporal gradient of

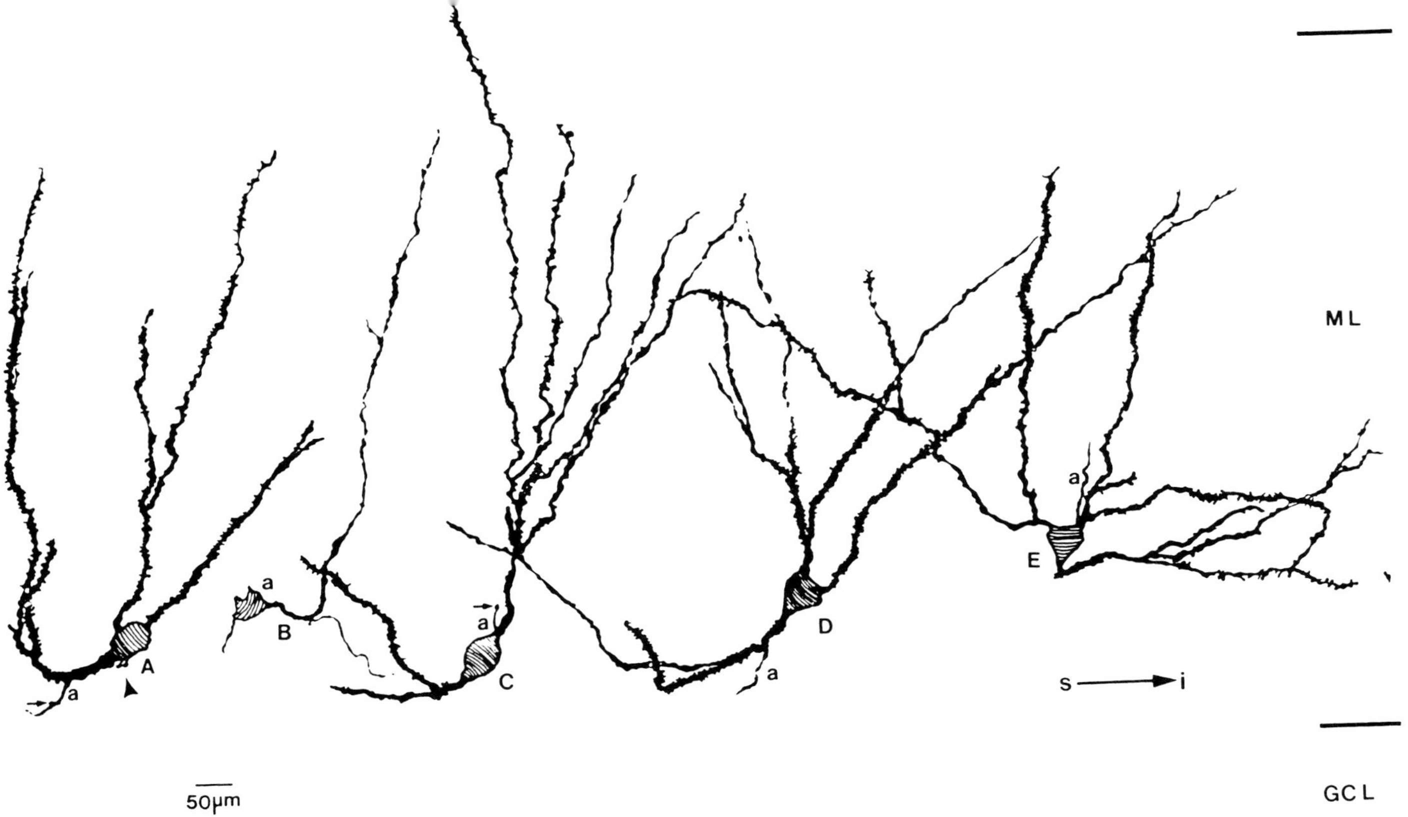

Figure 4.9. Camera-lucida drawings of Golgi-impregnated ectopic granule cells from the molecular layer of the dentate gyrus of NZB/BlNJ mice. The arrows point to bouton-like swellings on the axons. Abbreviations: a, axon; GCL, granule cell layer; ML, molecular layer, s→i, *supra*pyramidal-to-*infra*pyramidal spatiotemporal gradient.

cell birth indicates that *during development* the basally-directed dendritic processes are growing into an area occupied by processes from slightly more mature granule cells. The underlying assumption of these ideas is that the ectopic granule cells do not differ from their normally-positioned counterparts *intrinsically*; rather, any observed differences in their morphology are the result of environmental influences acting on them as a result of their ectopic position. The correlation of cell position and dendrite growth has been previously well-described for the molecular layer interneurons of the cerebellar cortex (Rakic, 1972, 1975). In the cerebellum the shape and form of the dendritic trees of these neurons is dependent on both the position of the cell body in the molecular layer *and* the interactions of the growing dendrites with the parallel fibers that comprise the bulk of the molecular layer. The 'rules' followed by the developing dendritic processes of the granule cells of the dentate gyrus appear to be identical to those followed by the molecular layer interneurons of the cerebellar cortex. In essence, a dendrite from either class of neuron proceeds as if it is maximizing the number of contacts it makes with its afferents. In the case of the cerebellum, the afferents to the molecular layer interneurons are the parallel fibers. In the case of the dentate gyrus, the afferents to the granule cells are the major axon systems (i.e. the commissural, associational, septal, entorhinal, etc.) of the molecular layer. The attractive feature of this idea is that it can also explain the differences between the upright, goblet shape of the dentate granule cells and the stellate shape of the cerebellar molecular layer interneurons. The explanation lies in the fact that the orientation of the individual axons comprising the afferent input to the dentate gyrus is more-or-less a series of columnar 'bouquets', while the afferent input in the cerebellum is that of parallel fibers organized tangential to the pial surface.

Relationship of immune dysfunction and neuronal migration

Recently, we have observed that four single autosomal mutations that are known to produce immune-system dysfunctions also have pleiotropic effects on neuronal migration during the development of the central nervous system (Nowakowski, 1988). Two of these mutants, motheaten (me^v/me^v) and beige (bg/bg) have similar disorders in the hippocampal formation and the cerebellar cortex (Fig. 4.10A, B). In the hippocampal formation of both motheaten and beige, a disruption of the migration of granule cells results in a trail of granule cells along the migratory route which extends from the ventricular zone to the dentate gyrus. Additional ectopic granule cells are located in the molecular layer of the dentate gyrus, and there are also ectopic pyramidal cells in the stratum oriens of area CA3. In the cerebellar cortex,

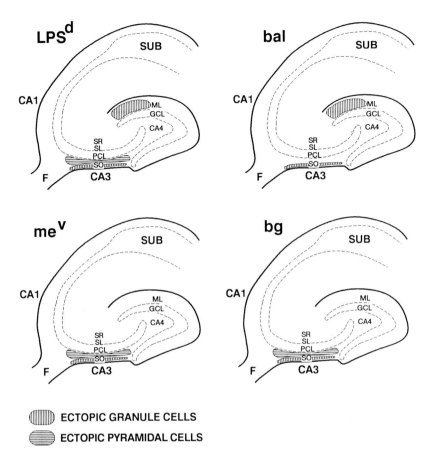

⬚ ECTOPIC GRANULE CELLS

≡ ECTOPIC PYRAMIDAL CELLS

Figure 4.10. Schematic drawings of the hippocampal formation of four mouse mutants that exhibit both immune-system dysfunctions and abnormalities in neuronal migration in the developing hippocampal formation: **LPS**^{d}, lipopolysaccharide response defect; **bal**, balding; **me**^{v}, motheaten viable; **bg**, beige. The general location of ectopic neurons in each of the four mutants is indicated by shaded area (see key). Abbreviations: F, fimbria; GCL, granule cell layer; ML, molecular layer; PCL, pyramidal cell layer; SL, stratum lucidum; SO, stratum oriens; SR, stratum radiatum; SUB, subiculum (Nowakowski, 1988).

islands of ectopic granule cells are located subpially, in the former position of the external granule cell layer. The other two mutants, lipopolysaccharide response defect (Lps^d/Lps^d) and balding (bal/bal), also have evidence of a disruption in the migration of granule cells in the hippocampal formation (Fig. 4.10C, D). The distribution of granule cells along the migratory pathway to the dentate gyrus is similar to that in the motheaten and beige mutations. However, there are no ectopic granule cells in the molecular layer, and the migration of granule cells in the cerebellar cortex does not appear to be adversely affected by these mutations. Ectopic pyramidal cells in area CA3, such as those found in motheaten and beige, are present in Lps^d but not in balding. Thus, four genetically distinct, single, autosomal mutations (three of which (me^v, bg, bal) arose spontaneously in the C57BL/6J inbred strain) produce phenotypically similar disruptions in neuronal migration during the development of the CNS. The immune dysfunctions of these four mutants are quite dissimilar (M. C. Green, 1981). Interestingly, neuronal migration in the hippocampal formation and the cerebellum appears normal in nude mice (nu/nu) which are genetically athymic. These results indicate that there is common gene expression during B cell differentiation and neuronal migration.

Genetic pleiotropism

Table 4.2 summarizes the effect of each of these mutations on the organization and development of the hippocampal region. The phenotypes resulting from these mutations range from a selective disruption of the migration of late-generated pyramidal cells to area CA3c to broadly distributed disruptions of cell position in all parts of the hippocampal formation. The dreher mutation seems to affect both cell proliferation and migration but not of all cell populations (Nowakowski & Wahlsten, 1985a,b). The reeler mutation affects the migration of all neurons but has minimal affects on cell number (Stanfield & Cowan, 1979a,b; Stanfield et al., 1979). In NZB/BlNJ mice it seems that migration of both pyramidal and granule cells is affected. The Hld mutation seems to affect the migration of only the late-generated pyramidal cells that are destined for area CA3c. The me^v and bg mutants affect both granule cells in the dentate gyrus and pyramidal cells in area CA3 of the hippocampus, while the bal and Lps^d mutations affect only the migration of the granule cells in the dentate gyrus. This variation in the effects of these mutations on the development of the hippocampal formation indicates that: (1) the mutant genes are probably expressed in different cell types; (2) the mutant genes are probably expressed at different times during development; and (3) a basic developmental process such as neuronal

88

Table 4.2. *The incidence of ectopic neurons in the hippocampal region and the cerebellar cortex in the eight mutants listed in Table 4.1. For details see text.*

Mutant	Granule cells of dentate gyrus in		Pyramidal cells of CA3 in		Layer I of entorhinal cortex	Granule cells in ML of cerebellar cortex
	ML	CA3	S.R.	S.O.		
dr^{sst-J}	+	+	+	+	+	+
Hld				+		+
rl^{Orl}				+	+	+
NZB	+			+	+	+
bal	+	+				
Lps^d	+	+				
me^v				+	+	+
bg				+	+	+

migration is influenced and perhaps controlled by a variety of cell–cell interactions that are functionally related to several different genes.

Table 4.2 also summarizes our observations on the distribution of the effects of each of these genes in other regions of the CNS, notably the cerebellum (Nowakowski, unpublished). For example, six of the mutations have ectopic pyramidal cells in area CA3; these same six mutations also have ectopic granule cells in the molecular layer of the cerebellar cortex. This association may reflect the existence of common gene expression during the migration of these two diverse cell types. The overlap in the phenotypes of the various mutations provides insight into the extent of common gene expression during neuronal migration.

Relevance to human disease

Neuronal migration and neuropathology

Neuronal migration has been implicated in a number of human diseases that affect cerebral cortical development and function, e.g. dyslexia (Galaburda, Sherman & Geschwind, 1983), autism (Bauman & Kemper, 1985), epilepsy (Meencke & Janz, 1984); thanatophoric dwarfism (Ho *et al.*, 1984); schizophrenia (Kovelman & Scheibel, 1984, 1986), fetal alcohol syndrome (Miller,

1986, 1989), radiation exposure (Otake & Schull, 1984), Fukuyama-type muscular dystrophy, and others (Evrard *et al.*, 1978; Choi & Kudo, 1981; Graff-Radford *et al.*, 1986; Galloway & Roessmann, 1987). The relationship of the developmental defects of the mutant mice being studied to human neuropathology may be of particular relevance with respect to the dysgenesis reported in dyslexia, epilepsy, thanatophoric dwarfism, and schizophrenia. Pathological reports for patients suffering from dyslexia, epilepsy and schizophrenia all describe islands of ectopic neurons in the hippocampus, neocortex and/or cerebellar cortex (Galaburda *et al.*, 1983; Meencke & Janz, 1984; Kovelman & Scheibel, 1984, 1986). These reports of microdysgenesis of cortical structures indicate that disruptions of neuronal migration have occurred during intrauterine life. The similarity of these human pathological descriptions to the malformations found in the mice being analyzed is striking. Also, the constellation of CNS and peripheral abnormalities (Ho *et al.*, 1984) and the incomplete recessiveness of thanatophoric dwarfism (McKusick, 1983) are similar to our findings for the dreher mouse (R. S. Nowakowski & D. Wahlsten, unpublished data).

TWO HIT HYPOTHESIS

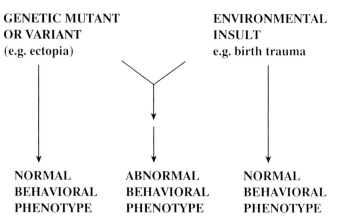

GENETIC MUTANT
OR VARIANT
(e.g. ectopia)

ENVIRONMENTAL
INSULT
e.g. birth trauma

NORMAL
BEHAVIORAL
PHENOTYPE

ABNORMAL
BEHAVIORAL
PHENOTYPE

NORMAL
BEHAVIORAL
PHENOTYPE

Figure 4.11. Schematic representation of the 'Two Hit Hypothesis' described in the text. This hypothesis is suggested to provide a biological basis for the inheritance of a predisposition or susceptibility to a late-onset disease. According to this hypothesis an abnormal behavioral phenotype may result from the additive effect of an otherwise non-deleterious genotype and an environmental event (or independent genotype) which also is relatively benign when both occur in the same organism. See text for further details. (Nowakowski, 1988.)

Two-hit hypothesis

Many neurological diseases, including such diverse disorders as Alzheimer's disease, multiple sclerosis, dyslexia and schizophrenia, are widely believed to have both genetic and environmental contributions to their etiology (e.g. Murray, Lewis & Reveley, 1985; Murray & Lewis, 1987; Martin, 1987). This idea stems from the observations that these and other neurological disorders occur more frequently in the siblings of an affected individual than in the general population, but as yet an obvious mode of inheritance (such as autosomal dominant or recessive) has not been demonstrated (McKusick, 1983). In the case of schizophrenia, there is a significant familial component and high (but not 100%) concordance in many twin studies (e.g. Crow *et al.*, 1989; Suddath *et al.*, 1990). The suggestion is, therefore, that people afflicted with such disorders have a genetic composition that *predisposes* them by providing a permissive arena for the action of some second event later in life.

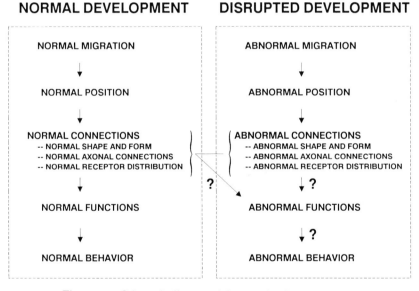

Figure 4.12. Schematic diagram of the cascade of events associated with normal and disrupted migration in the developing CNS. The diagram on the left shows the normal sequence of events, and the diagram on the right shows the disrupted sequence. If disruption of migration occurs in only one part of the CNS, the connections between the abnormally-positioned neurons and their normally-positioned counterparts may be affected, and abnormal functions and behaviour may result.

The genetic composition and the second, environmentally-related event (e.g. Mednick, this volume; Suddath *et al.*, 1990) are by themselves relatively benign, such that neither alone produces any overt pathology or behavioral change (Fig. 4.11). This idea is similar to the proposed two-hit models proposed for the genetic (somatic or germline) mutations that occur during oncogenesis (Land, Parada & Weinberg, 1983; Sinn *et al.*, 1987). In this context, the possibility of a 'family' of mouse mutations that affect the developing hippocampal region could be of great significance in understanding how such a two-hit hypothesis could contribute to the etiology of schizophrenia. The 'two-hit hypothesis' provides a convenient conceptual framework for dealing with the specific concept of an interaction of genetic and environmental components of schizophrenia, and with the more general concept of the inheritance of a predisposition. What remains to be elucidated, however, is the specific cascade of events (Fig. 4.12) that differs in normal and disrupted development of the CNS, and how normal and disrupted developmental processes coexist and interact in the same brain.

Acknowledgement

Supported by a grant from the Scottish Rite Schizophrenia Research Program.

References

Angevine, J. B., Jr (1965). Time of neuron origin in the hippocampal region: an autoradiographic study in the mouse. *Experimental Neurology Supplement*, **2**, 1–71.

Barber, R. P., Vaughn, J. E., Wimer, R. E. & Wimer, C. C. (1974). Genetically-associated variations in the distribution of dentate granule cell synapses upon the pyramidal cell dendrites in mouse hippocampus. *Journal of Comparative Neurology*, **156**, 417–34.

Bauman, M. & Kemper, T. L. (1985). Histoanatomic observations of the brain in early infantile autism. *Neurology*, **35**, 866–74.

Bayer, S. A. (1980*a*). Development of the hippocampal region in the rat. I. Neurogenesis examined with ^{3}H-thymidine autoradiography. *Journal of Comparative Neurology*, **190**, 87–114.

(1980*b*). Development of the hippocampal region in the rat. II. Morphogenesis during embryonic and early postnatal life. *Journal of Comparative Neurology*, **190**, 115–34.

Bayer, S. A., Yackel, J. W. & Puri, P. S. (1982). Neurons in the rat dentate gyrus granular layer substantially increase during juvenile and adult life. *Science*, **216**, 890–2.

Caviness, V. S., Jr (1973). Time of neuron origin in the hippocampus and dentate gyrus of normal and reeler mutant mice: an autoradiographic analysis. *Journal of Comparative Neurology*, **151**, 113–20.

(1982). Neocortical histogenesis in normal and reeler mice: a developmental study based upon [³H]thymidine autoradiography. *Developmental Brain Research*, **4**, 293–302.

Caviness, V. S. (1986). Genetic abnormalities of the developing nervous system. In A. K. Asbury, G. M. McKhann & W. I. McDonald (Eds.), *Diseases of the Nervous System* (pp. 22–35). Philadelphia: Saunders.

Caviness, V. S., Jr & Rakic, P. (1978). Mechanisms of cortical development: a view from mutations in mice. *Annual Review of Neuroscience*, **1**, 297–326.

Caviness, V. S., Jr & Sidman, R. L. (1973a). Retrohippocampal, hippocampal and related structures of the forebrain in the reeler mutant mouse. *Journal of Comparative Neurology*, **147**, 235–54.

(1973b). Time of origin of corresponding cell classes in the cerebral cortex of normal and reeler mutant mice: An autoradiographic analysis. *Journal of Comparative Neurology*, **148**, 141–52.

Choi, B. H. & Kudo, M. (1981). Abnormal migration and gliomatosis in epidermal nevus syndrome. *Acta Neuropathologica*, **53**, 319–25.

Cowan, W. M., Stanfield, B. B. & Kishi, K. (1980). The development of the dentate gyrus. *Current Topics in Developmental Biology*, **15**, 103–57.

Crow, T. J., Ball, J., Bloom, S. R., Brown, R., Bruton, C. J. & Colter, N. (1989). Schizophrenia as an anomaly of development of cerebral asymmetry: a postmortem study and a proposal concerning the genetic basis of the disease. *Archives of General Psychiatry*, **46**, 1145–50.

Eckenhoff, M. F. & Rakic, P. (1984). Radial organization of the hippocampal dentate gyrus: a Golgi, ultrastructural and immunocytochemical analysis in the developing rhesus monkey. *Journal of Comparative Neurology*, **223**, 1–21.

Evrard, P., Caviness, V. S., Jr, Prats-Vinas, J. & Lyon, G. (1978). The mechanism of arrest of neuronal migration in the Zellweger malformation: an hypothesis based upon cytoarchitectonic analysis. *Acta Neuropathologica*, **41**, 109–17.

Galaburda, A. M., Sherman, G. F. & Geschwind, N. (1983). Developmental dyslexia: third consecutive case with cortical anomalies. *Society for Neuroscience Abstracts*, **9**, 940.

Galloway, P. G. & Roessmann, U. (1987). Diffuse dysplasia of cerebral hemispheres in a fetus. Possible viral cause? *Archives of Pathology Laboratory Medicine*, **111**, 143–5.

Graff-Radford, N. R., Bosch, E. P., Stears, J. C. & Tranel, D. (1986). Developmental Foix–Chavany–Marie syndrome in identical twins. *Annals of Neurology*, **20**, 632–5.

Green, E. (1981). *Genetics and Probability in Animal Breeding Experiments*. New York: Macmillan.

Green, M. C. (1981). *Genetic Variants and Strains of the Laboratory Mouse*. Stuttgart: Gustav Fisher Verlag.

Herrup, K. (1983). Role of staggerer gene in determining cell number in cerebellar cortex. I. Granule cell death is an indirect consequence of staggerer gene action. *Brain Research*, **313**, 267–74.

Ho, K. L., Chang, C. H., Yang, S. S. & Chason, J. L. (1984). Neuropathologic findings in thanatophoric dysplasia. *Acta Neuropathologica (Berlin)*, **63**, 218–28.

Kaplan, M. S. & Hinds, J. W. (1977). Neurogenesis in the adult rat: electron microscopic analysis of light radioautographs. *Science*, **197**, 1092–4.

Kovelman, J. A. & Scheibel, A. B. (1984). A neurohistological correlate of schizophrenia. *Biological Psychiatry*, **19**, 1601–21.

(1986). Biological substrates of schizophrenia. *Acta Neurologica Scandinavica*, **73**, 1–32.

Land, H., Parada, L. F. & Weinberg, R. A. (1983). Cellular oncogenes and multistep carcinogenesis. *Science*, **222**, 771–8.

Lorente de No, R. (1934). Studies on the structure of the cerebral cortex. II. Continuation of the study of the ammonic system. *Journal für Psychologie und Neurologie*, **46**, 113–17.

Martin, J. B. (1987). Molecular genetics: Applications to the clinical neurosciences. *Science*, **238**, 765–77.

McKusick, V. A. (1983). *Mendelian Inheritance in Man*. Baltimore: Johns Hopkins University Press.

Meencke, H.-J. & Janz, D. (1984). Neuropathological findings in primary generalized epilepsy: a study of eight cases. *Epilepsia*, **25**, 8–21.

Miller, M. W. (1986). Effects of alcohol on the generation and migration of cerebral cortical neurons. *Science*, **233**, 1308–11.

(1989). Effect of prenatal exposure to ethanol on the development of the cerebral cortex: II. Cell proliferation in the ventricular and subventricular zones of the rat. *Journal of Comparative Neurology*, **287**, 326–38.

Mullen, R. & Herrup, J. (1979). Chimeric analysis of mouse cerebellar mutants, In X. O. Breakfield (Ed.), *Neurogenetics: Genetic Approaches to the Study of the Nervous System* (pp. 173–96). New York: Elsevier.

Murray, R. M. & Lewis, S. W. (1987). Is schizophrenia a neurodevelopmental disorder? *British Medical Journal*, **295**, 681–2.

Murray, R. M., Lewis, S. W. & Reveley, A. M. (1985). Towards an aetiological classification of schizophrenia. *Lancet*, **1(8436)**, 1023–6.

Nowakowski, R. S. (1984). The mode of inheritance of a defect in lamination in the hippocampus of the BALB/c mouse. *Journal of Neurogenetics*, **1**, 249–58.

(1985). Neuronal migration in the hippocampal lamination defect (Hld) mutant mouse. In H. J. Marthy (Ed.), *Cellular and Molecular Control of Direct Cell Interactions* (pp. 133–54). New York: Plenum Press.

(1986). Abnormalities in neuronal migration in the hippocampal formation of the NZB/BlNJ mouse. *Society for Neuroscience Abstracts*, **12**, 317.

(1988). Development of the hippocampal formation in mutant mice. *Drug Development Research*, **15**, 315–36.

Nowakowski, R. S. & Davis, T. L. (1985). Dendritic arbors and dendritic excrescences of abnormally positioned neurons in area CA3c of mice carrying the mutation 'hippocampal lamination defect'. *Journal of Comparative Neurology*, **239**, 267–75.

Nowakowski, R. S. & Rakic, P. (1979). The mode of migration of neurons to the hippocampus: A Golgi and electron microscopic analysis in the foetal rhesus monkey. *Journal of Neurocytology*, **8**, 697–718.

(1981). The site of origin and route and rate of migration of neurons to the hippocampal region of the rhesus monkey. *Journal of Comparative Neurology*, **196**, 129–54.

Nowakowski, R. S. & Wahlsten, D. (1985a). Anatomy and development of the hippocampus and dentate gyrus in the shaker short-tail (sst) mutant mouse. *Anatomical Record*, **211**, 140A.

(1985b). Asymmetric development of the hippocampal region in the shaker short-tail (sst) mutant mouse. *Society for Neuroscience Abstracts*, **11**, 989.

Otake, M. & Schull, W. J. (1984). In utero exposure to A-bomb radiation and mental retardation; a reassessment. *British Journal of Radiology*, **57**, 409–14.

Patrylo, P. R., Sekiguchi, M. & Nowakowski, R. S. (1990). Heterozygote effects in *dreher* mice. *Journal of Neurogenetics*, **6**, 173–81.

Pearlman, A. L. (1985). The visual cortex of the normal mouse and reeler mutant. In E. G. Jones & A. A. Peters (Eds.), *The Cerebral Cortex* (pp.1–18). New York: Plenum Press.

Rakic, P. (1972). Mode of cell migration to the superficial layers of fetal monkey neocortex. *Journal of Comparative Neurology*, **145**, 61–83.

(1975). Cell migration and neuronal ectopias in the brain. *Birth Defects: Original Article Series*, **11**, 95–129.

Rakic, P. & Nowakowski, R. S. (1981). The time of origin of neurons in the hippocampal region of the rhesus monkey. *Journal of Comparative Neurology*, **196**, 99–128.

Rickmann, M., Amaral, D. G. & Cowan, W. M. (1987). Organization of radial glial cells during the development of the rat dentate gyrus. *Journal of Comparative Neurology*, **264**, 449–79.

Schlessinger, A. R., Cowan, W. M. & Gottlieb, D. I. (1975). An autoradiographic study of the time of origin and the pattern of granule cell migration in the dentate gyrus of the rat. *Journal of Comparative Neurology*, **159**, 149–76.

Sherman, G. F., Galaburda, A. M. & Geschwind, N. (1985). Cortical anomalies in brains of New Zealand mice: a neuropathologic model of dyslexia. *Proceedings of the National Academy of Sciences, USA*, **82**, 8072–4.

Sidman, R. L., Angevine, J. B. & Taber-Pierce, E. (1971). *Atlas of the Mouse Brain and Spinal Cord*. Cambridge, Massachusetts: Harvard University Press.

Sinn, E., Muller, W., Pattengale, P., Tepler, I., Wallace, R. & Leder, P. (1987). Coexpression of MMTV/v-Ha-ras and MMTV/c-myc genes in transgenic mice: synergistic action of oncogenes in vivo. *Cell*, **49**, 465–75.

Staats, J. (1966). The laboratory mouse. In E. Green (Ed.), *Biology of the Laboratory Mouse* (pp. 1–9). New York: Dover.

Stanfield, B. B., Caviness, V. S., Jr & Cowan, W. M. (1979). The organization of certain afferents to the hippocampus and dentate gyrus in normal and reeler mice. *Journal of Comparative Neurology*, **185**, 461–84.

Stanfield, B. B. & Cowan, W. M. (1979a). The development of the hippocampus and dentate gyrus in normal and reeler mice. *Journal of Comparative Neurology*, **185**, 423–59.

(1979b). The morphology of the hippocampus and dentate gyrus in normal and reeler mice. *Journal of Comparative Neurology*, **185**, 393–422.

Suddath, R. L., Christison, G. W., Torrey, E. F., Casanova, M. F. & Weinberger, D. R. (1990). Anatomical abnormalities in the brains of monozygotic twins discordant for schizophrenia. *New England Journal of Medicine*, **322**, 791–4.

Vaughn, J. E., Matthews, D. A., Barber, R. P., Wimer, C. C. & Wimer, R. E. (1977). Genetically-associated variations in the development of hippocampal pyramidal neurons may produce differences in mossy fiber connectivity. *Journal of Comparative Neurology*, **173**, 41–52.

Wahlsten, D., Lyons, J. P. & Zagaja, W. (1983). Shaker short-tail, a spontaneous neurological mutant in the mouse. *Journal of Heredity*, **74**, 421–5.

Wyss, J. M. & Sripanidkulchai, B. (1985). The development of Ammon's horn and the fascia dentata in the cat: a ^{3}H-thymidine analysis. *Developmental Brain Research*, **18**, 185–98.

5

Is the genetic vulnerability to schizophrenia linked to abnormal development of the ventricular system and the brain barrier systems in the human fetal brain?

METTE STAGAARD, TORBEN MOOS AND
KJELD MØLLGÅRD

The Panum Institute, University of Copenhagen

Introduction

Several studies performed during the last decade have strongly indicated that heredity is of major importance in the etiology of schizophrenia (American Psychiatric Association, 1980; Lyon *et al.*, 1989). While the gene product is entirely unknown, genetic linkage analysis has provided data suggesting that genes on chromosome 5 and/or 19 may be involved in schizophrenia (Byerley *et al.*, 1989). According to a 'two-hit hypothesis', the genetic risk involves some unknown disturbance of the brain development, but additional environmental influences (exogenous factors) during gestation, or during the perinatal period, are required for later development of schizophrenia (Cannon, Mednick & Parnas, 1989). The genetic vulnerability of the developing brain could involve the brain *per se*: neuroepithelial cells, differentiating neurons and glial cells, and/or the interfaces between the brain and the outside world: the vascular system, the choroid plexuses, meninges, and circumventricular organs, i.e. the brain barrier systems.

Several exogenous factors have been proposed as candidates, e.g. emotional stress, radiation and viral infection during gestation, but perinatal complications are also likely to play a role in the later development of schizophrenia (Cannon *et al.*, 1989). Statistically, all of the exogenous factors may be involved, but virtually nothing is known about how or where their effects are exerted. Some exogenous factors may act in a more generalized 'unspecific' way involving all cells in the developing brain (e.g. highly lipid-soluble substances like anesthetics and alcohol), whereas other exogenous factors (e.g. protein molecules) may be specifically transported across the brain barriers or may circumvent the barriers via retrograde axonal transport and thus gain access to specific, localized areas of the brain.

The developing brain barrier systems

The developing brain barrier systems and the possible ways in which exogenous factors may enter the developing brain of the human fetus will be considered in the following. Exogenous factors may comprise well-known growth factors (e.g. NGF, EGF, PDGF, FGF; James & Bradshaw, 1984) and potential growth factors such as neurotransmitters, peptides and some plasma proteins, all of which are characterized by having specific targets or uptake and transport mechanisms (Pardridge, 1986). Plasma proteins are also transport molecules which carry biologically important material like hormones, vitamins or trace metals (e.g. iron, zinc, copper) but, unfortunately, also toxic substances which inadvertently may enter the brain (see below).

If the brain is not secluded from the outside world by functional brain barriers, or if the specific transcellular transport mechanisms carry unphysiological amounts of specifically wanted substances, then neuroepithelial cells as well as differentiating neurons and glial cells may receive wrong signals at a given time, perhaps resulting in premature cessation of mitosis, incomplete or inappropriate migration, incorrect positioning or, in the case of young neurons, formation of erroneous connectivity. At a given time in development the allocortex shows a marked difference compared to the neocortex in plasma protein distribution in the sheep (see figs. 12 A–D in Reynolds & Møllgård, 1985). Whether this difference reflects an increased receptor-mediated transport of plasma proteins across the blood–brain barrier of the allocortex or an increased plasma protein production by neurons in the developing human allocortex is now being investigated (Stagaard & Møllgård, unpublished).

Plasma proteins

Plasma proteins are well-known substances which are produced and secreted by the liver and circulate in the blood. Only few plasma proteins have documented functions of their own, like alpha–2–macroglobulin and alpha–1–antitrypsin, both of which are anti-proteolytic and present in high concentrations during pregnancy. Transferrin seems to be of particular importance for both the developing and adult brain. It has been shown to be an important constituent of defined media for the culture of nerve cells *in vitro*, where it appears to be associated with the growth of neurites (Bottenstein *et al.*, 1980; Skaper, Selak & Varon, 1982). So far it is not known whether the iron-carrying capability of transferrin is functionally important in the brain or whether transferrin has some other biological significance (Fishman *et al.*, 1987), e.g. a neuromodulatory function (Hill *et al.*, 1985).

From immunocytochemical studies it has been found that several plasma proteins are present within neurons and glial cells in the developing brain (Møllgård *et al.*, 1979). Immunochemical identification of proteins, which had been *in ovo* translated from specific mRNAs extracted from human fetal brain, has shown that proteins, which are indistinguishable from the plasma proteins produced in the liver, are also synthesized within the brain (Møllgård *et al.*, 1988). So far it has generally been assumed that plasma proteins are found in the fetal CSF because they penetrate a supposedly immature blood–brain barrier, but there is now very good evidence that the blood–brain barrier to proteins is well-formed even in the earliest stages of embryonic development and that major amounts of the intracerebral plasma proteins are derived from synthesis within the brain (c.f. Møllgård & Saunders, 1986; Møllgård *et al.*, 1988). Our current hypothesis is that the plasma proteins may be of functional significance for the differentiation of neurons and glial cells and for interactions between neuronal populations.

The brain barriers to plasma proteins and other macromolecules

The term 'blood–brain barrier' is used to describe a series of mechanisms that control the stability of the internal environment of the brain. These mechanisms include *impermeability* to large-molecular-weight solutes such as plasma proteins and protein-bound dyes, *limited permeability* to small-molecular-weight lipid insoluble molecules, and restricted transendothelial *receptor-mediated* transport. Due to the presence of specific enzymes within brain endothelial cells, various *metabolic* and *pharmacologic* barriers are operating. Finally, *specific efflux* mechanisms at the brain–blood interface are capable of moving solutes out of the brain against a concentration gradient. The effectiveness of all these barrier mechanisms is dependent on an underlying diffusion restriction, at the interface between the brain and the external environment, that is provided by tight junctions.

Tight junctions. Macromolecules including plasma proteins in the blood of adult mammals are largely excluded from the brain and cerebrospinal fluid (CSF) by the blood–brain, blood–CSF and pia-arachnoid–brain barriers

(Figs 5.1, 5.2A and B). Tight junctions between cerebral endothelial, choroid plexus epithelial, and pia-arachnoid cells constitute the morphological basis for these brain barrier systems (see, e.g., Brightman & Reese, 1969; Nabeshima et al., 1975).

As it is not possible to obtain evidence about the permeability of brain barriers in the human fetus by direct experimentation, indirect evidence has been obtained by studying the protein composition of human fetal CSF and the ultrastructure of barriers in the developing human brain. Serial thin sections and freeze-fracture replicas, prepared from 16 embryonic and fetal brains, have shown that the characteristic appearance of tight junctions is present between cerebral endothelial cells, choroid plexus epithelial cells and pia-arachnoid cells as early as week 7 of gestation (Møllgård & Saunders, 1986, and unpublished results). The rather limited data from human fetuses have been compared with results from various animal experiments and the comparison suggests that information obtained from experimental fetal animals is, to a large extent, of value in interpreting the state of the human brain barrier development.

Neuroepithelial strap junctions and the ventricular system. In the adult vertebrate CNS, the brain interstitial fluid and CSF are in continuity and both contain low concentrations of proteins (Davson, Welch & Segal, 1987). However, fetal CSF has a high protein content (Dziegielewska & Saunders, 1988) and is isolated from brain interstitial fluid by a new fourth barrier with an ultrastructural appearance different from that of the above-mentioned 'tight junction' barriers. This new barrier, which was first described in the developing *sheep* brain (Møllgård et al., 1987) is located to the ventricular zone (Fig. 5.3); it consists of 'strap junctions' between adjacent neuroepithelial cells. The strap junctions are single-stranded membrane specializations arranged in a spiralled fashion from the ventricular pole of the cells along the lateral cell membrane towards the subventricular zone. These junctions form the morphological basis for a CSF–brain barrier to protein found in early, but not in late, fetal sheep brain (Fossan et al., 1985; Møllgård et al., 1987).

In the developing *human* brain these junctions become less prominent at week 16 of gestation. At about week 22 of gestation the neuroepithelial cells of the ventricular zone are gradually replaced by a mature-looking ependymal cell layer in which the individual cells are connected by large gap junctions, while neither tight nor strap junctions are present. The presence of junctions between neuroepithelial cells in the germinal matrix appears to account for the observations that macromolecules including plasma proteins are not present in the extracellular space of early human fetal brains (unpublished

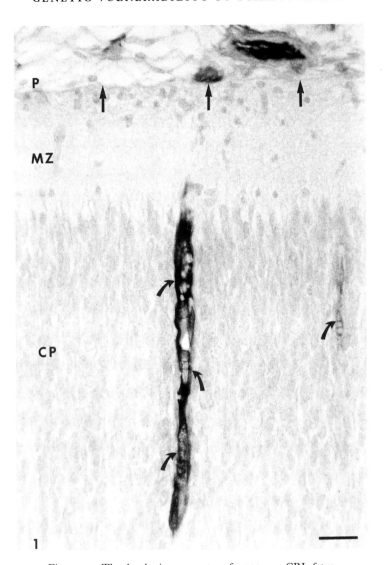

Figure 5.1. The developing neocortex of a 109-mm CRL fetus is devoid of alpha-fetoprotein immunoreactivity, except for the intravascular staining. The interface between vascular wall and brain (curved arrows) indicate the presence of a tight blood–brain barrier. A barrier is also present at the brain and pia-arachnoid (P) interface (long arrows). The section has been counterstained with toluidine blue. MZ, marginal zone; CP, cortical plate. Bar: 50 μm.

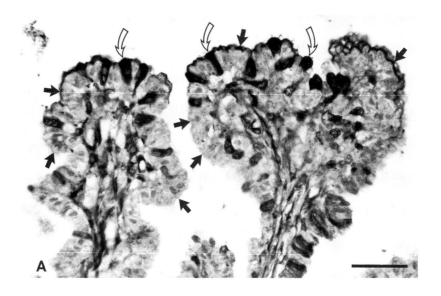

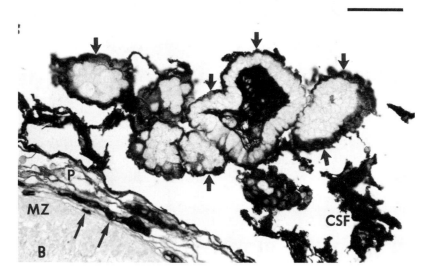

Figure 5.2 (A and B). Choroid plexus from fourth ventricle of a
38 mm CRL embryo, immunostained for alpha–2–HS
glycoprotein (A), and a 123-mm CRL fetus immunostained for
albumin, with toluidine blue counterstaining (B). Short arrows
indicate the interface between the CSF and the choroid plexus,
which represents the blood–CSF barrier. Single cells exhibit
intense intracellular reaction for plasma protein (A: open
curved arrows) which is transcytosed from blood to CSF.
Although the choroid plexus epithelial cells in B are devoid of
reaction, the presence of a reaction product on either side of

data). As the ventricular strap junctions gradually disappear during development, the concentration of the CSF-protein declines in parallel. Therefore, in the developing brain it seems that presumptive neurons are only exposed to a high external protein concentration at early stages of their development, namely when they are differentiating within the germinal matrix and still have part of their cell surface in contact with the protein-rich CSF.

One possible explanation for this compartmentalization is that the ventricular zone, which is the primary source of dividing and migrating neurons and glia, bordering the CSF could need a 'high-protein medium' to stimulate proliferation, whereas a low protein concentration is required in the brain interstitial fluid so that specific proteins produced by neurons and glial cells might act as effective local growth factors, morphogens and signals. Effective ion regulation of the interstitial fluid and CSF appears relatively late in development (Jones & Keep, 1987), presumably correlated with the maturation of excitability mechanisms and integrated synaptic activity. Thus, cell layers acting as diffusion barriers in the fetal brain seem to be designed to segregate proteins in different compartments, suggesting that the most important extracellular signals in developing brain are proteins rather than small ions.

Communication between the external environment and the brain

Over the last 15 years, receptor-mediated endocytosis has been recognized as the mechanism by which mammalian cells specifically internalize macromolecules (for review see Goldstein et al., 1985). Receptor-mediated endocytosis applies to many transport plasma proteins (e.g. transferrin and albumin) as well as to non-transport plasma proteins including asialoglycoproteins, alpha–2–macroglobulin, and immune complexes. Certain viruses and toxins use receptor-mediated endocytosis to enter cells, apparently by binding opportunistically to receptors that normally function in the uptake of other substances. Protein growth factors, such as epidermal growth factor (EGF) and platelet-derived growth factor (PDGF), as well as classic polypeptide hormones, such as insulin and luteinizing hormone, also enter cells by receptor-mediated endocytosis (c.f. Goldstein et al., 1985).

Receptor-mediated endocytosis from the luminal side of endothelial or epithelial cells followed by transcellular transport and exocytosis from the abluminal side is referred to as receptor-mediated transcytosis (Pardridge,

Caption for fig. 5.2 (cont.)
the cells and in CSF precipitate within the ventricle (B: CSF) suggest that transport across the brain–CSF barrier is taking place. The interface between the brain parenchyma and the pia-arachnoid is indicated by long arrows (B). MZ, marginal zone; P, pia-arachnoid. Bar: 50 μm.

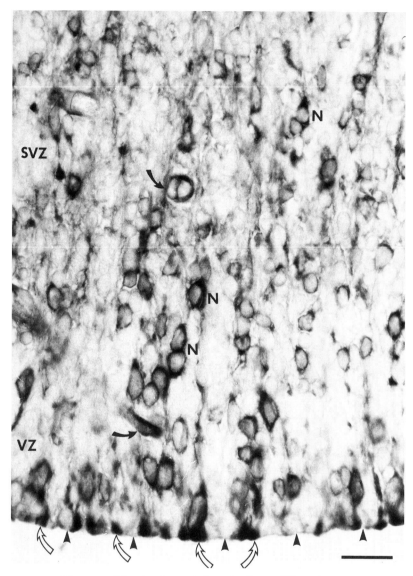

Figure 5.3. The rhombencephalon of a 28-mm CRL embryo has been immunostained for albumin. The interface between the brain parenchyma and the CSF (the CSF–brain barrier) exhibits no intercellular staining, but alternating cells are seen to have (open curved arrows) or not to have (arrowheads) endocytosed the plasma protein from the CSF. In the brain, migrating young neurons (N) are albumin positive. The interface between blood and brain, i.e. the blood–brain barrier, is shown by curved arrows. VZ: ventricular zone. SVZ: subventricular zone. Bar: 20 μm.

1986). Non-selective fluid phase endocytosis may also lead to (non-specific) transcytosis (of, e.g., horseradish peroxidase (HRP)) but this process is insignificant or does nor occur in the brain (Balin *et al.*, 1986).

The blood–brain barrier. The initial statement that brain capillary endothelial cells have a paucity of pinocytotic vesicles was based on HRP-injection experiments; thus it was a question of relatively few HRP-containing vesicles in gray matter of adult mouse parietal cortex (Reese & Karnovsky, 1967). Conventional thin-section electron microscopy of rat *allocortex, brainstem, and cerebellum* reveals that brain capillary endothelium in many regions exhibits membrane specializations and membranous compartments which may be associated with receptor-mediated endocytosis and transcytosis (Møllgård, Balslev & Saunders, 1988). These include invaginations at the luminal surface, coated and uncoated vesicular profiles, endosome- and lysosome-like bodies including multivesicular bodies, and also vesicles in contact with the abluminal surface.

The finding of transferrin receptors located specifically to endothelium of brain capillaries (Jefferies *et al.*, 1984) was the first indication that endogenous proteins cross the blood–brain barrier by receptor-mediated endocytosis. Pardridge (1986) has more recently summarized evidence for the presence of at least five peptide receptors (including transferrin) on cerebral capillaries, and developed the concept that transport systems for peptides, like transport systems for nutrients, exist on the blood–brain barrier and mediate uptake of circulating peptides. Endogenous albumin and transferrin have been detected in vesicular and tubular profiles of brainstem endothelial cells, suggesting that not only transferrin but also albumin is transported via a receptor (Møllgård *et al.*, 1988). The existence of albumin receptors on continuous visceral capillary endothelia has previously been described (Ghitescu *et al.*, 1986).

The choroid plexus and the blood–CSF barrier. So far there is no evidence to indicate that receptors specific for plasma proteins exist on the plasmalemma of choroid plexus epithelial cells, but in a recent investigation (Møllgård & Balslev, 1989) transferrin and albumin were found inside a membranous system, which resemble the transepithelial IgG-transport system which has been described in newborn rat ileum (Rodewald & Abrahamson, 1982). Receptors for peptides and transmitter substances have been shown (Davson *et al.*, 1987), but a specific transepithelial transport system has not been demonstrated.

The pia-arachnoid–brain and the (fetal) CSF–brain barrier. Receptor-mediated transcytosis across these barriers has not been described so far, but the ultrastructure of the cell layers involved suggest that this may in fact occur.

Retrograde axonal transport from the external environment. The brain barrier systems can be circumvented by transport via axons from motor neurons in the spinal cord and cranial nerve nuclei in the brainstem which project to the periphery (the external environment). Due to both receptor-mediated uptake and fluid phase endocytosis followed by retrograde axonal transport, substances such as viruses, bacterial toxins, dye–protein complexes and heavy metals that are introduced into or present in the external environment can later be detected in the neuronal perikarya (for references see Møllgård & Saunders, 1986). Furthermore, findings of Behnsen (1927) and Kristensson, Olsson & Sjöstrand (1971) also seem to indicate that retrograde axonal transport is even more prominent in neonatal than in adult mice, possibly because the endocytosis by unmyelinated growing axon terminals is more pronounced (Møllgård & Saunders, 1986).

Some brain regions, the circumventricular organs, act as 'windows' of contact between the brain and the external environment, as originally observed by Behnsen (1927). These organs, which comprise median eminence, neurohypophysis, pineal gland, organum vasculosum laminae terminalis, subfornical organ and area postrema, lie adjacent to the median ventricular cavities. They all possess fenestrated capillaries, resulting in an absence of a blood–brain barrier in the organ *per se* but, instead, a presence of a blood–CSF barrier localized between the specialized ependymal cells (Brightman, Prescott & Reese, 1975). Thus, substances circulating in the blood gain entrance to these restricted areas of the brain (Kristensson *et al.*, 1971; Schultzberg *et al.*, 1988), permitting signals from the outside to exert their effects either locally or via retrograde axonal transport at distant target neurons which project to the circumventricular organs. Exogenous substances may then be taken up in projecting axons via receptor-mediated or fluid-phase endocytosis in axon terminals and transported to neuronal perikarya inside the blood–brain barrier, e.g. via projections from the supraoptic and paraventricular nuclei to the neurohypophysis, a pathway that is normally involved in the secretion of vasopressin and oxytocin.

Conclusion

Regions originally developed from the medial telencephalic wall – hippocampus, dentate gyrus, parahippocampus, amygdala and septal area – seem to be the areas of primary concern in the neuropathology of schizophrenia (Bogerts, Meerts & Schonfeld-Bausch, 1985; Falkai & Bogerts, 1986; Falkai,

Bogerts & Rozumek, 1988; Jakob & Beckmann, 1986; Kovelman & Scheibel, 1984). Areas which are also affected, but not directly linked to the hippocampal formation, include the dorsomedial thalamic nucleus (Pakkenberg & Gundersen, 1988), the prefrontal cortex (Andreasen *et al.*, 1986; Weinberger, Berman & Zec, 1986), the basal ganglia (Bogerts *et al.*, 1985; including nucleus accumbens: B. Pakkenberg, personal communication) and the vermis (Heath, Franklin & Shraberg, 1979). Enlargement of the third and lateral ventricles is a consistent finding in adult schizophrenics (Weinberger, Wagner & Wyatt, 1983), which is also found in non-affected monozygotic twins (Reveley *et al.*, 1982).

Exogenous factors

Exogenous factors, for example lipid-soluble molecules, which will gain access to the entire brain irrespective of the presence of functional barriers, could cause a *generalized* damage of the proliferative zones of the developing brain, resulting in premature cessation of mitosis, cell deficiency and ventricular enlargement. Such factors are, however, unlikely to be responsible for the localized neuropathological changes found in schizophrenia. The dominating feature of embryonic and early fetal brain is a state of physiological hydrocephalus. If the ventricular cells of the proliferative zones are damaged, the hydrocephalus may become even more pronounced, and the protein concentration of the brain interstitial fluid may be elevated because of inadequate function of the strap junctions. Interestingly, the heavy metal tellurium administered to pregnant rats on gestational days 10–15 has been shown to cause fatal hydrocephalus in neonatal rats, the mechanism of which is unknown (see Adams, Corsellis & Duchen, 1984, pp. 260–303, 451–90, 627–98).

The localized brain regions and exogenous factors

Exogenous factors capable of producing *localized* damage may in principle gain access to the interior of the brain by four mechanisms: (1) specific exogenous factor combined with specific transport; (2) unspecific exogenous factor combined with specific transport; (3) specific exogenous factor combined with unspecific transport; (4) specific or unspecific exogenous factor combined with specific blood–brain barrier breakdown.

(1) A given transport plasma protein (e.g. albumin) carrying fatty acids, testosterone, estradiol or thyroid hormone, may be endocytosed and

recycled, while the ligand gains access to the brain via receptor-mediated transcytosis across blood–brain or blood–CSF barriers. Alternatively, it may have gained access via retrograde axonal transport.

(2) The same plasma protein now carrying, e.g., toxic heavy metals like lead or aluminium in addition to a physiological ligand, will be transported as above, but the unwanted substance will have gained access as well.

(3) Certain viruses and toxins apparently bind opportunistically to re-ceptors that normally function in the uptake of other substances, and are endocytosed and possibly transcytosed (Goldstein et al., 1985). Alternatively, the substance may enter via fluid-phase endocytosis followed by transcytosis or retrograde axonal transport.

(4) Plasma proteins, heavy metals, viruses or toxins will enter at localized sites in the brain when the blood–brain barrier is subjected to unphysiological challenges.

Studies on the maturity and effectiveness of the barrier systems have indicated that there is some reproducibility in the localization of the ensuing affected sites and presumptive leakages. This may explain why various neurological diseases with a wide range of etiological agents exhibit a remarkably uniform pattern of localized neuropathological changes. The hippocampal formation, and in particular Ammon's horn, is a much-preferred target of a number of severe conditions, e.g. infection with herpes simplex virus and rabies; chronic intoxication with lead, trimethyl tin and bismuth; and in kuru and kernicterus. Thalamus and vermis are other frequently affected regions in infections and intoxication as well as in kernicterus (see Adams et al., 1984).

Receptor-mediated endocytosis and heredity

The genetic vulnerability to schizophrenia may be caused by deficient receptor-mediated transport across the brain barrier systems. A comparison can be based on the molecular biological findings in the familial form of hypercholesterolemia, the etiology of which was recently elucidated (Brown & Goldstein, 1984). This disease, which results in severe atherosclerosis, has been shown to be caused by genetic defects in the receptor for plasma low-density liproprotein (LDL). A number of different, naturally-occurring mutations result in lack of receptor function which precludes cellular uptake of LDL via receptor-mediated endocytosis (c.f. Goldstein et al., 1985). In the developing human brain there is some indication that receptor-mediated transport of plasma protein is more pronounced in the hippocampal formation than, e.g., in the neocortex (unpublished data). This would seem logical as this region is known to contain large amounts of zinc, which must be delivered specifically by the alpha–2–zinc binding globulin, or by one of three other plasma proteins with known zinc-binding properties: albumin, alpha–2–macroglobulin, and transferrin (Shaw, 1979). For each of these proteins there are known or proposed receptors on the endothelial cells. In analogy with the genetic defects in the LDL receptor, we suggest that a defect in the proposed alpha–2–zinc binding globulin receptor will cause zinc deficiency inside the hippocampal formation with altered cell proliferation and differentiation (Warkany & Petering, 1972). Furthermore it is conceivable that a reduced zinc supply may trigger or stimulate other zinc-transporting systems. A resulting increased activity of receptor-mediated uptake of, e.g., zinc–albumin complexes may lead to concomitant uptake of hormones, vitamins, fatty acids or noxious substances (see mechanism (2) in the previous section). Other brain regions affected in schizophrenia may also be characterized by a high content of heavy metals, e.g. iron in the basal ganglia, and are therefore dependent on uptake via transferrin receptors. A genetic defect in these receptors could result in similar disturbances. Since the developing human brain is also synthesizing plasma proteins (Møllgård et al., 1988), which may handle the intracerebral transport of zinc, iron and other potentially toxic heavy metals, we find it attractive to investigate the distribution of plasma proteins inside the hippocampal formation and its microvasculature in the developing human brain from control and high-risk fetuses. Such investigations are in progress.

Acknowledgements

We wish to thank Keld Bo Ottesen for excellent technical assistance. The study is supported by A. & A.D. Bjørnmoses Mindelegat.

References

Adams, J. H., Corsellis, J. A. N. & Duchen, L. W. (Eds.) (1984). *Greenfield's Neuropathology* (4th edn.). London: Edward Arnold.
American Psychiatric Association. (1980). DSM-III: *Diagnostic and Statistical Manual of Mental Disorders*. (3rd edn.) Washington: American Psychiatric Association.
Andreasen, N. C., Nasrallah, H. A., Dunn, V., Olson, S. C., Grove, W. M., Ehrhardt, J. C., Coffman, J. A. & Crossett, J. H. W. (1986). Structural abnormalities in the frontal system in schizophrenia. *Archives of General Psychiatry*, **43**, 136–44.
Balin, J. B., Broadwell, R. D., Salcman, M. & El-Kalliny, M. (1986). Avenues for

entry of peripherally administered protein to the central nervous system in mouse, rat, and squirrel monkey. *Journal of Comparative Neurology*, **251**, 260–80.

Behnsen, G. (1927). Über die Farbstoffspeicherung in Zentralnervensystem der Weissen Maus in Verschiedenen Alterszuständen. *Zeitschrift für Zellforschung und mikroskopische Anatomie*, **4**, 515–72.

Bogerts, B., Meerts, E. & Schonfeld-Bausch, R. (1985). Basal ganglia and limbic system pathology in schizophrenia. *Archives of General Psychiatry*, **42**, 784–91.

Bottenstein, J. F., Skaper, S. D., Varon, S. S. & Sato, G. H. (1980). Selective survival of neuron from chick embryo sensory ganglionic dissociates utilizing serum-free supplemented medium. *Experimental Cell Research*, **125**, 183–90.

Brightman, M. W., Prescott, L. & Reese, T. S. (1975). Intercellular junctions of special ependyma. *Brain–Endocrine Interaction II*. Basel: Karger.

Brightman, M. W. & Reese, T. S. (1969). Junctions between intimately apposed cell membranes in the vertebrate brain. *Journal of Cell Biology*, **40**, 648–77.

Brown, M. S. & Goldstein, J. L. (1984). How LDL receptors influence cholesterol and atherosclerosis. *Scientific American*, **251**, 58–61.

Byerley, W., Mellon, C., O'Connell, P., Lalouel, J.-M., Nakumura, Y., Leppert, M. & White, R. (1989). Mapping genes for manic-depression and schizophrenia with DNA markers. *Trends in Neurosciences*, **12**, 46–8.

Cannon, T. D., Mednick, S. A. & Parnas, J. (1989). Genetic and perinatal determinants of structural brain deficits in schizophrenia. *Archives of General Psychiatry*, **46**, 883–9.

Davson, H., Welch, K. & Segal, M. B. (1987). *Physiology and Pathophysiology of the Cerebrospinal Fluid*. Edinburgh: Churchill Livingstone.

Dziegielewska, K. M. & Saunders, N. R. (1988). The development of the blood–brain barrier: Proteins in fetal and neonatal CSF, their nature and origins. In E. Meisami & P. J. Timira (Eds.), *Handbook of Human Growth and Biological Development*. Bora Raton: CRC Press.

Falkai, P. & Bogerts, B. (1986). Cell loss in the hippocampus of schizophrenics. *European Archives of Psychiatry and Neurological Sciences*, **236**, 154–61.

Falkai, P., Bogerts, B. & Rozumek, M. (1988). Limbic pathology in schizophrenia: The entorhinal region – a morphometric study. *Biological Psychiatry*, **24**, 515–21.

Fishman, J. B., Rubin, J. B., Handrahan, J. V., Connor, J. R. & Fine, R. E. (1987). Receptor-mediated transcytosis of transferrin across the blood–brain barrier. *Journal of Neuroscience Methods*, **18**, 299–304.

Fossan, G., Cavanagh, M. E., Evans, C. A. N., Malinowska, D. H., Møllgård, K., Reynolds, M. L. & Saunders, N. R. (1985). CSF–brain permeability in the immature sheep fetus: A CSF–brain barrier. *Developmental Brain Research*, **18**, 113–24.

Ghitescu, L., Fixman, A., Simionescu, M. & Simionescu, N. (1986). Specific binding sites for albumin restricted to plasmalemmal vesicles of continuous capillary endothelium: Receptor-mediated transcytosis. *Journal of Cell Biology*, **102**, 1304–11.

Goldstein, J. L., Brown, M. S., Anderson, R. G. W., Russell, D. W. & Schneider, W. J. (1985). Receptor-mediated endocytosis: concepts emerging from the LDL receptor system. *Annual Review of Cell Biology*, **1**, 1–39.

Heath, R. G., Franklin, D. E. & Shraberg, D. (1979). Gross pathology of the cerebellum in patients diagnosed and treated as psychiatric disorders. *Journal of Nervous and Mental Disease*, **167**, 585–92.

Hill, J. M., Ruff, M. R., Weber, R. J. & Pert, C. B. (1985). Transferrin receptors in rat brain: Neuropeptide-like pattern and relationship to iron distribution. *Proceedings of the National Academy of Sciences, USA*, **82**, 4553–7.

Jakob, H. & Beckmann, H. (1986). Prenatal development disturbances in the limbic allocortex in schizophrenics. *Journal of Neural Transmission*, **65**, 303–26.

James, R. & Bradshaw, R. A. (1984). Polypeptide growth factors. *Annual Reviews of Biochemistry*, **53**, 259–92.

Jefferies, W. S., Brandon, M. R., Hunt, S. V., Williams, A. F., Gatter, K. C. & Mason, D. Y. (1984). Transferrin receptor on endothelium of brain capillaries. *Nature, London*, **312**, 162–3.

Jones, H. C. & Keep, R. F. (1987). The control of potassium concentration in the cerebrospinal fluid and brain interstitial fluid of developing rats. *Journal of Physiology, London*, **383**, 441–53.

Kovelman, J. A. & Scheibel, A. B. (1984). A neurohistological correlate of schizophrenia. *Biological Psychiatry*, **19**, 1601–21.

Kristensson, K., Olsson, Y. & Sjöstrand, J. (1971). Axonal uptake and retrograde transport of exogenous proteins in the hypoglossal nerve. *Brain Research*, **32**, 399–406.

Lyon, M., Barr, E. C., Cannon, T. D., Mednick, S. A. & Shore, D. (1989). Fetal neural development and schizophrenia. *Schizophrenia Bulletin*, **15**, 149–61.

Møllgård, K. & Balslev, Y. (1989). The subcellular distribution of transferrin in rat choroid plexus studied with immunogold labelling of ultracryosections. *Histochemical Journal* (1989). **21**, 441–8.

Møllgård, K., Balslev, Y., Lauritzen, B. & Saunders, N. R. (1987). Cell junctions and membrane specializations in the ventricular zone (germinal matrix) of the developing sheep brain: a CSF–brain barrier. *Journal of Neurocytology*, **16**, 433–44.

Møllgård, K., Balslev, Y. & Saunders, N. R. (1988). Structural aspects of the blood–brain and blood–CSF barriers with respect to endogenous proteins. In L. Rakic, H. Davson, D. J. Begley & B. V. Zlokovic (Eds.), *Peptide and amino acid transport mechanisms in the central nervous system* (pp. 93–101). London and Belgrade: Macmillan Press and Serbian Academy of Science and Arts.

Møllgård, K., Dziegielewska, K. M., Saunders, N. R., Zakut, H. & Soreq, H. (1988). Synthesis and localization of plasma proteins in the developing human brain: Integrity of the fetal blood–brain barrier to endogenous proteins of hepatic origin. *Developmental Biology*, **128**, 207–21.

Møllgård, K., Jacobsen, M., Jacobsen, G. K., Clausen, P. P. & Saunders, N. R. (1979). Immunohistochemical evidence for an intracellular localization of plasma proteins in human fetal choroid plexus and brain. *Neuroscience Letters*, **14**, 85–90.

Møllgård, K. & Saunders, N. R. (1986). Annotation: The development of the human blood–brain and blood–CSF barriers. *Neuropathology and Applied Neurobiology*, **12**, 337–58.

Nabeshima, S., Reese, T. S., Landis, D. M. D. & Brightman, M. W. (1975). Junctions in the meninges and marginal glia. *Journal of Comparative Neurology*, **164**, 127–70.

Pakkenberg, B. & Gundersen, H. J. G. (1988). Total number of neurons and glial cells in human brain nuclei estimated by the dissector and the fractionator. *Journal of Microscopy*, **150**, 1–20.

Pardridge, W. M. (1986). Receptor-mediated peptide transport through the blood–brain barrier. *Endocrine Reviews*, **7**, 314–30.

Reese, T. S. & Karnovsky, M. J. (1967). Fine structural localization of a blood–brain barrier to exogenous peroxidase. *Journal of Cell Biology*, **34**, 207–17.

Reveley, A. M., Reveley, M. A., Clifford, C. H. & Murray, R. M. (1982). Cerebral ventricular size in twins discordant for schizophrenia. *Lancet*, **6**, 540–1.

Reynolds, M. L. & Møllgård, K. (1985). The early distribution of plasma proteins in the neocortex and early allocortex of the developing sheep brain. *Anatomy and Embryology*, **171**, 41–60.

Rodewald, R. & Abrahamson, D. R. (1982). Receptor-mediated transport of IgG across the intestinal epithelium of the neonatal rat. *Ciba Foundation Symposium*, **92**, 209–32.

Schultzberg, M., Ambatsis, M., Samuelson, E.-B., Kristensson, K. & van Meirvenne, N. (1988). Spread of *Trypanosoma brucei* to the nervous system: Attack on circumventricular organs and sensory ganglia. *Journal of Neuroscience Research*, **21**, 56–61.

Shaw, J. C. L. (1979). Trace elements in the foetus and young infant. I. Zinc. *American Journal of Diseases in Children*, **133**, 1260–8.

Skaper, S. D., Selak, J. & Varon, S. S. (1982). Molecular requirements for survival of cultured avian and rodent dorsal root ganglionic neurons responding to different trophic factors. *Journal of Neuroscience*, **8**, 251–61.

Warkany, J. & Petering, H. G. (1972). Congenital malformations of the central nervous system in rats produced by maternal zinc. *Teratology*, **5**, 319–34.

Weinberger, D. R., Berman, K. F. & Zec, R. F. (1986). Physiologic dysfunction of dorsolateral prefrontal cortex in schizophrenia: I. Regional cerebral blood flow evidence. *Archives of General Psychiatry*, **43**, 114–24.

Weinberger, D. R., Wagner, R. L. & Wyatt, R. J. (1983). Neuropathological studies of schizophrenia: a selective review. *Schizophrenia Bulletin*, **9**, 193–212.

Part IV

Genetic and teratogenic disturbances in the etiology of schizophrenia

6

Obstetrical events and adult schizophrenia

SARNOFF A. MEDNICK, TYRONE D. CANNON AND
CHRISTOPHER E. BARR

University of Southern California

In this chapter we consider the evidence that obstetrical complications (OCs) are of etiological significance in schizophrenia. We first consider three etiological models that might include a role for OCs.

Model 1: OCs as the sole cause of schizophrenia

Given the demonstrated importance of genetic factors in schizophrenia, OCs could only be the 'sole' cause of schizophrenia if they were the phenotypic expression of the genetic predisposition. With this formulation the genetic condition would predispose to serious OCs; serious OCs would be sufficient to cause schizophrenia. This possibility seems very unlikely. Too many infants who do not become schizophrenic are born with OCs just as severe as any observed in schizophrenics. This explanation also fails to explain the sizable subgroup of schizophrenics who have apparently not experienced severe OCs (Cannon, Mednick & Parnas, 1990a; Cannon, Mednick & Parnas, 1990b). In addition, this model is discredited by individuals at high genetic risk for schizophrenia who do not suffer exceptional levels of OCs.

Model 2: OCs as the sole cause for SOME schizophrenics

It has been suggested that some cases of schizophrenia are caused solely or mainly by genetic factors while other cases are caused solely or mainly by OCs (Lewis & Murray, 1987). This hypothesis has grown from the results of some studies which have reported that schizophrenics with a familial psychiatric history evidence no OCs, while those schizophrenics with OCs evidence no family history of mental illness (Cazullo, Vita & Sacchetti, 1989; Schwarzkopf et al., 1989; Reveley, Reveley & Murray, 1984).

These studies may have a methodological weakness; the obstetrical history and the family psychiatric history are usually obtained by interview with parents of the adult schizophrenic. The parent is asked to recall pregnancy and delivery events which occurred 20–30 years before. Aside from the fact that the parent (usually the mother) is hardly an objective observer, the problem of separating this child's OCs from those of the other children in the family, and the substantial amount of time elapsed since the event, may make this method of data acquisition less than ideal (Mednick & Shaffer, 1963; Mednick & Hefner, 1969). This fact has not escaped Murray and his colleagues (Murray, Reveley & Lewis, 1988). Murray is also aware of the fact that some families try to develop a theory to explain why their child became schizophrenic. One possible family theory might involve a psychotic grandparent and purposefully exclude other interpretations; another family might concentrate upon a complicated pregnancy and delivery.

In addition to these conceptual problems, McNeil (1988) has demonstrated empirically that parental recall of the obstetrical history of their adult psychiatrically-hospitalized children is woefully incomplete. Murray has countered that perhaps only the important OCs remain in recall after 20–30 years and that this may be an advantage. Be that as it may, most of us (including Murray) would very likely be more convinced by prospective data gathered by professionals at the time of the pregnancy and delivery.

It should be pointed out that genetic factors may not be suited to be a sole cause of schizophrenia, even for a subgroup of schizophrenics. Many identical twins are discordant for schizophrenia. Some environmental factors must combine or interact with genetic predisposition to increase the risk for the affected twins (Gottesman & Shields, 1982).

Given these considerations, it is difficult to see how either genetics alone or OCs alone could be responsible for schizophrenia.

Model 3: Genetic–OC interaction as cause of some cases of schizophrenia

This two-factor-interaction approach handles some of the logical difficulties mentioned above. It suggests that a genetically-provoked vulnerability of the fetus makes it especially susceptible to damage from OCs. According to this model, an infant who has a strong genetic predisposition and suffers severe OCs has a very high risk of succumbing to schizophrenia. (We do not mean to

Table 6.1. *Results of studies comparing obstetrical complication rates of childhood psychotics and normal subjects*

Study	Affected group	Type of complications
Mura (1974)	Childhood psychotics	More PCs and DCs
Taft & Goldfarb (1964)	Childhood psychotics	More PCs and DCs
Vorster (1960)	Childhood psychotics	More PCs and DCs
Knobloch & Pasamanick (1962)	Childhood psychotics	More PCs and DCs
Whittam, Simon & Mittler (1966)	Childhood psychotics	More DCs
Bender (1973)	Childhood psychotics	More DCs
Rutt & Offord (1971)	Childhood psychotics	More DCs
Hinton (1963)	Childhood psychotics	More PCs
Torrey & Hersch (1975)	Childhood psychotics	More PCs
Zitrin, Ferber & Cohen (1964)	No difference	
Terris, LaPouse & Monk (1964)	No difference	

suggest that this causal pattern fits all schizophrenics. See Cannon, Mednick & Parnas, in 1990b.) This is a view we favor; it will be developed and specified below.

Evidence for excessive OCs in schizophrenics

The literature relating to the obstetrical experiences of schizophrenics has been examined in 1978 and 1988 by Thomas McNeil. He has provided the field with thoughtful and complete reviews. McNeil's reviews (McNeil, 1988; McNeil & Kaij, 1978) give us the luxury of presenting a brief summary and proceeding to our interpretation of the findings.

OCs in childhood psychotics and autistic children

It is not certain that these studies of childhood psychotics are relevant to adult schizophrenia. It should be recalled, however, that a large percentage of childhood psychotics later manifest schizophrenia as adults. Table 6.1 summarizes the results of the 11 studies we found in the literature. Nearly all of the studies relied on parent interview for the OC information. As we

117

indicated earlier, this poses certain methodological difficulties. These parental reports, however, were often supplemented by birth certificates or hospital records. These studies are consistent in finding a higher level of OCs in the childhood psychotics than in the controls. The first four studies in Table 6.1 found a significant excess of both pregnancy (PCs) and delivery complications (DCs). The next three studies report significantly more delivery complications while the Hinton (1963) and Torrey & Hersch (1975) studies only found an excess of pregnancy complications. Terris, LaPouse & Monk (1964) and Zitrin, Ferber & Cohen (1964) observed no significant differences; the data for these last two studies were restricted to birth certificates. Gittleman & Birch (1967), examined IQ in a sample of childhood schizophrenics and noted that those with OCs had a significantly lower IQ.

A recent study of autistic children noted that they were characterized by an abnormality of the vermis which the authors attribute to a failure of fetal neural development due to genetic or teratogenic influences during the pregnancy (Courchesne et al., 1988).

In summary, there is a preponderance of evidence indicating that childhood psychosis is associated with an excessive level of OCs.

OCs in adult schizophrenics

Table 6.2 lists the studies which ascertained OCs for adult schizophrenics and controls. Katz (1939) examined the birth records for 100 individuals suffering schizophrenia and dementia praecox (who were described as evidencing 'progressive mental deterioration') as well as 100 matched controls. Katz reported significantly more OCs for the schizophrenics. The schizophrenics evidenced significantly more prematurity and had suffered a longer labor. The Woerner, Pollack & Klein (1971) study is of interest since it utilized two sibling control groups, abnormal and normal sibs. The schizophrenics had significantly more OCs than their normal siblings but not significantly more than their abnormal siblings. The Lane & Albee (1966) and second study by Woerner et al. (Woerner, Pollack & Klein, 1973) also utilized sibling controls, both finding that the birth certificates of the schizophrenics showed them to have been six ounces lighter at birth than their sibs. The study by Pollack et al. (1966) found no difference between the schizophrenics and their sibs. Their data source, however, was maternal interviews.

The three Scandinavian studies (Parnas et al., 1982; McNeil & Kaij, 1978; and Jacobsen & Kinney, 1980) utilized hospital and midwife records of OCs produced at the time of the pregnancy and delivery. All three show the schizophrenics as having suffered more frequent and more severe OCs than

Table 6.2. *Results of studies comparing obstetrical complication rates of schizophrenics and normal subjects*

Study	N	Findings
Katz (1939)	100 schizophrenics	Schizophrenics: more OCs
	100 controls	
Parnas et al. (1982)	12 schizophrenics	Schizophrenics: worse OCs
	25 schizotypals	Schizotypals: least OCs
	55 high risk controls	
McNeil & Kaij (1978)	54 process schizophrenics	Process schiz.: more PCs & DCs
	46 psychotics	
	100 controls	
Jacobsen & Kinney (1980)	63 schizophrenics	Schizophrenics: more frequent & severe DCs
	63 controls	
Lewis & Murray (1987)	955 psychiatric patients	Schizophrenics: more OCs than other psychiatric patients
Lane & Albee (1966)	52 schizophrenics	Schizophrenics: lower birth weight
	115 siblings	
Woerner et al. (1971)	34 schizophrenics	Schizophrenics: lower birth weight
	42 siblings	
Woerner et al. (1973)	46 schizophrenics	Schizophrenics: more PCs & DCs than normal siblings
	37 normal siblings	
	17 abnormal siblings	
Pollack et al. (1966)	33 schizophrenics	No difference
	33 siblings	

controls. The large study by Lewis & Murray (1987) found that the mothers of the schizophrenics report a greater frequency of OCs than do the mothers of other psychiatric patients.

To date, four studies have been conducted that investigate the relationship between exposure to a major influenza epidemic during fetal development and later rates of adult schizophrenia. The first study examined the aftermath of the 1957 Type A2 influenza epidemic in Helsinki (Mednick *et al.*, 1988). Those exposed to the epidemic during their second trimester of fetal development had significantly increased rates of schizophrenia. This result held independently for males and females, and in each of the several mental hospitals in greater Helsinki. The association was found for schizophrenia and not other mental illnesses.

Barr, Mednick & Munk-Jorgensen (1990) analyzed a data set consisting of the following information for each of the 480 months from 1910–1950: (1) the number of people born in Denmark; (2) the number of those born each month who later were diagnosed schizophrenic in a Danish psychiatric hospital; (3) the number of cases of influenza reported to the Danish Ministry of Health in each month; (4) the population of Denmark during this 40-year period.

The data set includes over 7500 schizophrenics; this makes it possible to examine a window of vulnerability somewhat narrower than a trimester. Barr *et al.* (1990) noted that unusually high levels of influenza occurring during the 6th and 7th months of gestation were associated with unusually high rates of future adult schizophrenics being born.

Since the Helsinki study, Torrey, Rawlings & Waldman (1988) examined the relationship between fetal exposure to viral infection and adult schizophrenia in Connecticut and Massachusetts, with inconsistent results. One possible reason for these mixed results was that Torrey *et al.* could not determine the place of birth of their samples. Given the immigration and mobility rates in the United States, some considerable number of their schizophrenics (perhaps 50%) were very likely born in states or nations other than Connecticut or Massachusetts; for such subjects, the viral disease frequencies and timing data for the states of Massachusetts and Connecticut may be irrelevant. The results of this study must be viewed with considerable caution.

Kendell & Kemp (1989) report a significant increase in adult schizophrenia for Edinburgh residents who were exposed to the 1957 influenza epidemic during month 6 of gestation. The number of cases for this finding is rather small, however, (five index and one control). Kendell & Kemp also report on the rates of adult schizophrenia for all of those in Scotland who were exposed to the 1957 epidemic. Unfortunately, their data suffer from the same problem as the Torrey *et al.* (1988) data set; they do not have information on place of birth of their subjects. In addition they point out that a large number of

Scottish males emigrated during the period of the study and may have been diagnosed schizophrenic in other countries. The data for the females is, therefore, more reliable. From data presented by Kendell & Kemp for Scotland (their Table 3), we examined the rates of adult schizophrenia (number of female adult schizophrenics per 1000 live-born females) for each trimester of exposure to the 1957 influenza epidemic. The schizophrenia rates for exposure in first, second and third trimesters, respectively, were 1.62, 2.70, and 1.28, per 1000 live-born Scottish females. Females exposed in the second trimester evidenced a significantly greater rate of schizophrenia than females exposed in the first or third trimesters (Chi square (2) = 7.23, $p < 0.01$). In view of the difficulties with this data set, this finding must be interpreted with caution.

Kendell & Kemp (1989) also point out that there were very severe influenza epidemics in 1918 and 1919; they reason that they would expect to see corresponding elevations in the rates of schizophrenia among those who, as fetuses, were exposed to these epidemics. They use a Scottish national psychiatric register for this study. Unfortunately, this register does not include the date of birth of the schizophrenics. It only includes the schizophrenics' statements of age at time of admission. Based on inspection of the data (rather than statistical analysis), they concluded there is no increase in births of future schizophrenics in 1918 and 1919. We completed a trend analysis of the data they present in their Table 3 and find a significant increase in birthrate of schizophrenics for 1919.

It is difficult to determine the implications of the Torrey *et al.* (1988) study for the viral hypothesis of schizophrenia because of the serious problems in their data sources. The Kendell & Kemp data (as analyzed above) do offer modest support for the viral hypothesis. The Finnish and Danish studies may be interpreted as suggesting that disturbances in fetal neural development may increase the risk of adult schizophrenia.

Twin studies

The study of the case histories of monozygotic (MZ) twins discordant for schizophrenia enables us to isolate environmental factors which may be involved in the etiology of schizophrenia. This strategy has been used to examine OC differences within monozygotic twin pairs. The twin pairs share many delivery conditions, although the first-born twin typically suffers fewer DCs. One twin usually has a lower birth weight. Table 6.3 summarizes the findings of these studies. All of the twin studies listed in Table 6.3 utilized maternal interview as their source of OC information.

Pollin & Stabenau (1968) noted that the schizophrenic twin of the pair had

121

Table 6.3. *Results of studies comparing obstetrical complication rates of schizophrenics and their co-twins*

Study	N	Findings
Pollin & Stabeneau (1968)	100 discordant MZ twins	Schizophrenic twin: lower birth weight
Gottesman & Shields (1972)	82 discordant twin pairs	No difference
McNeil & Kaij (1978)	39 discordant twin pairs	Schizophrenic twin: more DC's
Revely *et al.* (1983)	21 schizophrenic MZ pairs 18 MZ controls	Schizophrenics with family history: No OCs. Schizophrenics: fewer OCs than controls

a significantly lower birth weight. Gottesman & Shields (1972) reported no difference in birth weight. McNeil & Kaij (1978) reexamined the Gottesman & Shields data and noted a significantly higher level of DCs for the schizophrenic twin. Reveley *et al.* (1984) found that if a schizophrenic twin pair reported a familial psychiatric history they tended to report a surprisingly low level of OCs. The Reveley *et al.* (1984) study supports a replacement theory: that is, schizophrenia is caused by genetics in some cases and by OCs in the other cases. It should be emphasized that several studies have not found a dissociation between OCs and family history (McNeil, 1988).

Individuals at high risk for schizophrenia

Systematic studies of children at high risk for schizophrenia began in the early 1960s in an attempt to observe and record characteristics of schizophrenics before their special life conditions (drug treatment, failures, long-term hospitalization, isolation, etc.) obscured their premorbid characteristics and warped the memories of their experiences. One other important advantage of high-risk studies was noted in a recent review of this area of research: 'If a low-risk control group is included in the design, then it is possible to evaluate whether a given environmental stressor affects the HR and LR groups differently. In other words the design encourages the examination of gene–environment interactions in the etiology of the illness.' (Mednick & Silverton, 1988, p. 544). If such an interaction were discovered, careful study may shed light on the nature of the biological phenotypic expression of the genetic predisposition for schizophrenia.

There have been a number of reports that have noted interaction effects involving genetic predisposition for schizophrenia and OCs. The first of these reports was presented at a meeting of the Society for Social Biology. Mednick *et al.* (1971) studied the pregnancies and deliveries of all the children born to schizophrenic parents ($N = 83$) in a total Copenhagen birth cohort that had been the subject of an intensive perinatal investigation. They note that 'low birth weight in the children born to schizophrenics is associated with developmental abnormalities in their one-year examination. Children born with identical low birth weights in the other two (Control) groups show no evidence of such effects at one year' (Mednick et al., 1971, p. 112). At this same meeting Heston and Fish (Fish, 1971) offered another interpretation. They suggested that the developmental retardation and the eventual schizophrenia were both produced by the same genetic condition; the low birth weight was simply another manifestation of genetically-determined growth retardation. The high-risk method offers a test of the differences in interpretation of these findings.

If genetic factors are responsible for the obstetrical problems (such as low birth weight) as well as the developmental retardation in the high-risk group then we would hypothesize that high-risk offspring, being at higher genetic risk, would experience a higher level of OCs than controls. If the occurrence of OCs is independent of genetic background for schizophrenia, then high-risk subjects would not necessarily be expected to evidence elevated levels of OCs.

The two reviews by McNeil (McNeil & Kaij, 1978; McNeil, 1988) have examined the research relating to this question and concluded that there is no evidence of a higher level of OCs among high-risk offspring than among low-risk offspring. This absence of a difference has been noted in many studies (Mirdal *et al.*, 1974; Marcus *et al.*, 1981; Hanson, Gottesman & Heston, 1976). (There are a few reports, however, of increased anomalies for high-risk subjects during gestation. These will be discussed below and in the chapters on pregnancy.) The evidence favors the interpretation that OCs are not significantly elevated among those at genetically-defined high risk for schizophrenia, suggesting that the interaction interpretation may be more viable.

This type of interaction of genetic strain with perinatal complications has been reported in the animal genetic literature. Ingalls *et al.* (1953) found that strains of mice differ in the probability of litters suffering a genetically-determined sternum malformation. Under normal conditions, strain DBA/1 has a probability of 0.05, while strain C57B4/cd has a probability of 0.30 of developing sternum malformations. If the pregnancy of the mother mouse is disturbed by subjecting her to five hours of low atmospheric pressure on day 9 of pregnancy, the probability of the malformation increases. The DBA/1 strain has an increase of 70%; the C57B4/cd strain has an increase of 15%. The same pregnancy stress has dramatically different effects on the mice as a function of their genetic background. Note also that there is a genetic predisposition to the malformation and an independent predisposition to malformations resulting from the pregnancy stress!

Another instance of a gene–perinatal interaction was noted by Rieder, Broman & Rosenthal (1977). These investigators examined the perinatal records and IQ test scores (at age seven) of subjects in the Boston sample of the Collaborative Study of Mental Retardation and Cerebral Palsy (Broman, Nichols & Kennedy, 1975). They identified the schizophrenic parents in the cohort, and correlated obstetrical events with the IQ test scores for both the high-risk and low-risk subjects. Vaginal bleeding, edema and conduction anesthesia explained 34% of the variance in IQ scores in the offspring of 'continuous schizophrenics' (i.e. chronic, borderline and chronic schizoaffective schizophrenics, $N = 45$); The obstetrical factors did not relate to IQ in the controls or in a group with acute schizophrenia in their parents. The authors point out that it is possible to interpret these results as showing that a common genetic liability is responsible for the obstetrical complications, IQ deficit, and schizophrenia. This interpretation, however, would require that high-risk children have a lower IQ than low-risk children. This has not been observed (Mednick & Schulsinger, 1965). As Reider et al. (1977, p. 799) state, the interaction interpretation better explains their findings: 'children of schizophrenics are specifically susceptible to certain perinatal events . . .'

Marcus et al. (1981) studied the perinatal history and neurointegrative functioning of 58 Jerusalem-born high-risk infants. They found that, in 'every case, low to low-normal birth weight in an infant of a schizophrenic was associated with poor performance during the first year' (Marcus et al., 1981, p. 710). No such relationship was observed in the controls. The authors suggest the 'hypothesis of a genetically determined vulnerability of fetal brains of offspring of schizophrenics'.

The Copenhagen high-risk study has followed a group of 207 high-risk and 104 low-risk subjects for the past 26 years. In 1972, 15 of the high-risk offspring were diagnosed schizophrenic (Schulsinger, 1976). These 15 schizophrenics had significantly elevated levels of perinatal complications. It is significant that low-risk subjects with equivalent levels of perinatal complications did not evidence schizophrenia (Parnas et al., 1982).

As mentioned earlier, the high-risk subjects who had become schizophrenic evidenced significantly wider third ventricles and larger

124

ventricle–brain ratios than non-schizophrenic high-risk subjects. Furthermore, obstetrical complications were significantly related to third ventricle width and ventricle–brain ratios (Schulsinger *et al.*, 1984), and the interaction between degree of genetic risk and birth complications accounted for 56% of the variance in the ventricular measurements (Cannon, Mednick & Parnas, 1989).

The results of these varied studies offer encouraging evidence for the hypothesis that the high-risk fetus has a special vulnerability to neurological sequelae as a result of perinatal complications.

Our interpretation of these data

In this review we have noted several strands of evidence which implicate a disturbance in fetal neural development in the etiology of adult schizophrenia.

(1) Finnish and Danish epidemiological studies suggest that a disruption of the growth of the fetal brain in the second trimester may increase the risk for schizophrenia.

(2) We have noted that low birth weight and prematurity at birth are characteristic of schizophrenics and of the affected members of monozygotic twins discordant for schizophrenia. These findings imply that some disturbance during the gestation of schizophrenics interferes with normal growth.

(3) The elevated frequency of minor physical anomalies in schizophrenics may be interpreted as indicating genetic or teratogenic disturbances during gestation.'

(4) Recent neuropathological findings in schizophrenics have been interpreted as being caused by disruptions in neuronal migration, perhaps in the second trimester of gestation.

The origin of the hypothesized neural developmental disturbance may be genetic. Genetic factors can distort the organization of brain structures or functional systems by producing perturbations in the generation or migration of young neurons. Genetic factors have been found to be quite potent in producing such defects in laboratory animals (Nowakowski, 1987).

Models of adult syndromes of schizophrenia

We hypothesize that fetal neural developmental disturbance may be a critical part of the phenotypic expression of the genetic predisposition to schizophrenia. A teratogenic agent (such as a viral infection) striking during a critical period of brain development might mimic the genetic influence.

Some of those with the genetic predisposition who suffer the fetal developmental disruption may experience severe delivery complications. Our review has noted an elevation of delivery complications for a subgroup of schizophrenics. In our high-risk project we also noted a significant elevation of delivery complications among the schizophrenics (Fig. 6.1). But about half of the schizophrenics had no complications or very minor complications. This is reflected in the high level of delivery-complication score variance in the schizophrenics. Those high-risk subjects who had suffered severe delivery complications evidenced large ventricle–brain ratios and widening of their third ventricles (Cannon *et al.*, 1989; Silverton *et al.*, 1985) and evidenced a significantly increased risk for schizophrenia with predominantly negative symptoms (Cannon, Mednick & Parnas, 1990b). This suggests that delivery complications and enlarged ventricles may be involved in the etiology of a particular subgroup of schizophrenics. We have conducted several analyses of the Copenhagen high-risk project data bank in order to characterize the nature of this subgroup.

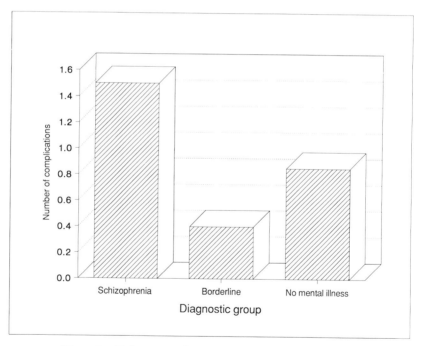

Figure 6.1. Delivery complications in high-risk subjects diagnosed as schizophrenic, borderline schizophrenic (SPD), and non-mentally-ill.

Third ventricle widening attracted our special attention since it is the most commonly reported CT-scan anomaly in schizophrenics and because of our long interest in the role of the autonomic nervous system in the etiology of schizophrenia (Mednick, 1985). The most important excitatory centers of the autonomic nervous sytem border on the third ventricle (Wang, 1964; Barr, 1979). We hypothesized that widening of the third ventricle is associated with damage to one or more of these autonomic nervous system centers. We have found that widening of the third ventricle is significantly associated with non-responding of the autonomic nervous sytem, both for electrodermal and heart-rate responsiveness (Cannon et al., 1988; Cannon, et al., in press). (This association is independent of the size of the lateral cerebral ventricles.)

We have suggested that perhaps damage to these excitatory autonomic nervous system centers (such as the anterior hypothalamus) may seriously dampen sympathetic nervous system activity and result in deficient emotional and motivational responsiveness. A non-responsive autonomic nervous system may contribute to anergia, often a part of the pattern of negative symptoms observed in schizophrenics.

This series of findings and interpretations led us to the prediction that genetic risk, delivery complications and autonomic nervous system non-responsiveness increase the risk for schizophrenia with predominantly negative symptoms.

We tested this model in the data of the Copenhagen high-risk study. In 1972 we diagnosed 15 schizophrenics. On the basis of the interview data, we prepared standardized scales measuring degree of negative and positive symptoms in the high-risk sample. We noted seven schizophrenics with severe negative symptoms and weak or absent positive symptoms. We tested the three hypothesized factors (genetic risk, severe delivery complications autonomic nervous system non-responding) to see how well they distinguished these seven negative-symptom schizophrenics from the other high-risk subjects. The genetic risk variable was expressed at two levels: super-high risk (schizophrenic mother and schizophrenia-spectrum father), and high risk (schizophrenic mother only).

Fig. 6.2 shows a decision-tree model test of this hypothesis. The rate of predominantly negative-symptom schizophrenia in the high-risk sample is 4%. If the individual is at super-high risk (i.e. has a spectrum father) the rate of negative-symptom schizophrenia increases to 11%. If the individual has experienced above-average delivery complications then the rate of negative-symptom schizophrenia is 35%. If (in 1962) these individuals were also autonomic nervous system non-responders, the rate of negative-symptom schizophrenia is 86%! Note that 131 high-risk subjects (including 8 schizophrenics with dominant positive symptoms) are classified by this

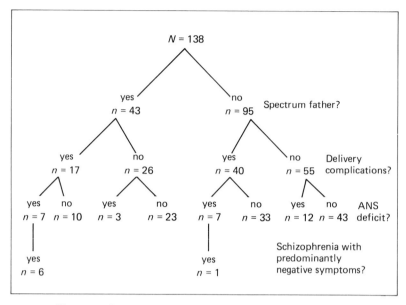

Figure 6.2. Decision-tree model of the etiology of schizophrenia with predominantly negative symptoms. (From Cannon, Mednick & Parnas, 1990b.)

model as *not* having negative-symptom schizophrenia. Only one of these 131 cases is misclassified.

In this framework, super-high risk status implies an extremely high risk that a genetically-determined disruption in fetal neural development occurred during the second trimester of gestation. We have found possible signs of this disruption of development in specific defects in cognitive performance which distinguish the super-high risk from the high-risk and low-risk subjects. (These defects include signs noted by Fini Schulsinger when the subjects were first interviewed in 1962; clouded consciousness, incoherence, disorientation, and impaired train of associations, as well as indices of word association disturbance and poor performance on standardized IQ tests.) We propose that the developmental disruption which may be responsible for these cognitive deficits is part of the etiological background of schizotypal personality disorder, a condition genetically related to schizophrenia. We have proposed in an earlier paper that schizotypal personality disorder is the basic 'genetic' disorder of the schizophrenia spectrum. In this framework, schizophrenia-proper is a derivative condition whose likelihood is increased by the action of certain environmental agents (such as OCs).

Summary

(1) The evidence strongly supports the role of OCs in the etiology of schizophrenia.

(2) The weight of the evidence indicates that OCs are most strongly associated with schizophrenia in individuals at high genetic risk.

(3) Epidemiological and neuropathological studies suggest that the phenotypic expression of the genetic predisposition for schizophrenia may consist of a disruption of brain development during gestation.

(4) In genetically vulnerable individuals, OCs increase the risk for periventricular tissue damage and later schizophrenia.

(5) The genetics–OCs interaction may help to explain schizophrenia with predominantly negative symptoms (and weak or absent positive symptoms).

Acknowledgements

This research was supported by National Institute of Mental Health Grants 5RO1 MH37692-04, 5RO1 MH37692-05, 2RO1 MH41469-04, a National Research Service Award from the National Institute of Mental Health to T. D. Cannon, and a Grant from the Scottish Rite Foundation.

References

Barr, M. L. (1979). *The human nervous system* (3rd edn). Hagerstown, Maryland: Harper & Row.

Barr, C. E., Mednick, S. A. & Munk-Jorgensen, P. (1990). Exposure to influenza epidemics during gestation and adult schizophrenia: A 40 year study. *Archives of General Psychiatry*, **47**, 869–74.

Bender, L. (1973). The life of course of children with schizophrenia. *American Journal of Psychiatry*, **130**, 783–6.

Broman, S. H., Nichols, P. I. & Kennedy, W. A. (Eds.). (1975). *Preschool IQ: Prenatal and Early Developmental Correlates*. New York: Halstead Press.

Cannon, T. D., Fuhrmann, M., Mednick, S. A., Machon, R. A., Parnas, J. & Schulsinger, F. (1988). Third ventricle enlargement and reduced electrodermal responsiveness. *Psychophysiology*, **25**, 153–6.

Cannon, T. D., Mednick, S. A. & Parnas, J. (1989). Genetic and perinatal determinants of structural brain abnormalities in schizophrenia. *Archives of General Psychiatry*, **46**, 883–9.

Cannon, T. D., Mednick, S. A. & Parnas, J. (1990a). Two pathways to schizophrenia in children at risk. In L. Robins & M. Rutter (Eds.), *Straight and devious pathways from childhood to adulthood*. (pp. 328–50). Cambridge: Cambridge University Press.

129

Cannon, T.D., Mednick, S.A. & Parnas, J. (1990b). Antecedents of predominantly negative and predominantly positive symptom schizophrenia in a high-risk population. *Archives of General Psychiatry*, **47**, 622–32.

Cannon, T.D., Raine, A., Herman, T.M., Mednick, S.A., Parnas, J. & Schulsinger, F. (1990). Third ventricle enlargement and reduced heart rate levels in a high-risk sample. *Psychophysiology*, in press.

Cazullo, C.L., Vita, A. & Sacchetti, E. (1989). Cerebral ventricular enlargement in schizophrenia: Prevalence and correlates. In S.C. Schulz & C.A. Tamminga (Eds.), *Schizophrenia: Scientific progress*. (pp. 195–206). New York: Oxford University Press.

Courchesne, E., Yeung-Courchesne, R., Press, G.A., Hesselink, J.R. & Jernigan, T.L. (1988). Hypoplasia of cerebellar vermal lobules VI and VII in autism. *New England Journal of Medicine*, **318**, 1349–54.

Fish, B. (1971). Genetic or traumatic developmental deviation. *Social Biology*, **18**, 117.

Gittleman, M. & Birch, H.G. (1967). Childhood schizophrenia: intellect, neurologic status, perinatal risk, prognosis, and family pathology. *Archives of General Psychiatry*, **17**, 16–25.

Gottesman, I.I. & Shields, J. (1972). *Schizophrenia and genetics: A twin study vantage point*. New York: Academic Press.

Gottesman, I.I. & Shields, J. (1982). *Schizophrenia: The epigenetic puzzle*. Cambridge: Cambridge University Press.

Hanson, D.R., Gottesman, I.I. & Heston, L.L. (1976). Some possible childhood indicators of adult schizophrenia inferred from children of schizophrenics. *British Journal of Psychiatry*, **129**, 142.

Hinton, G.G. (1963). Childhood psychosis or mental retardation: A diagnostic dilemma. II. Paediatric and neurological aspects. *Canadian Medical Association*, **89**, 1020–4.

Ingalls, T.H., Avis, F.R., Curley, F.G. & Temim, H.M. (1953). Genetic determinants of hypoxia-induced congenital anomalies. *Journal of Heredity*, **44**, 185–94.

Jacobsen, B. & Kinney, D.K. (1980). Perinatal complications in adopted and non-adopted schizophrenics and their controls: preliminary results. *Acta Psychiatrica Scandinavica Supplement*, **285**(62), 337–51.

Katz, B. (1939). *The etiology of the deteriorating psychoses of adolescence and early adult life*. Unpublished doctoral dissertation, University of Southern California.

Kendell, R.E. & Kemp, I.W. (1989). Maternal influenza in the etiology of schizophrenia. *Archives of General Psychiatry*, **46**, 878–82.

Knobloch, H. & Pasamanick, B. (1962, September). *Etiologic factors in 'early infantile autism' and 'childhood schizophrenia'*. Paper presented at the 10th International Congress of Paediatry, Lisbon.

Lane, E.A. & Albee, G.W. (1966). Comparative birth weights of schizophrenics and their siblings. *Journal of Psychology*, **64**, 227–31.

Lewis, S.W. & Murray, R.M. (1987). Obstetric complications, neurodevelopmental deviance, and risk of schizophrenia. *Journal of Psychiatric Research*, **21**, 413–21.

Marcus, J., Auerback, J., Wilkinson, L. & Burack, C. M. (1981). Infants at risk for schizophrenia. The Jerusalem Infant Development Study. *Archives of General Psychiatry*, **38**, 703–13.

Marcus, J., Hans, S. L., Mednick, S. A., Schulsinger, F. & Michelsen, N. (1985). Neurological dysfunctioning in offspring of schizophrenics in Israel and Denmark: A replication analysis. *Archives of General Psychiatry*, **42**, 753–61.

McNeil, T. F. (1988). Obstetric factors, and perinatal injuries. Obstetric factors and perinatal injuries. In M. T. Tsuang & J. C. Simpson (Eds.), *Handbook of schizophrenia* (pp. 319–44). Amsterdam: Elsevier.

McNeil, T. F. & Kaij, L. (1978). Obstetric factors in the development of schizophrenia: Complications in the births of preschizophrenics and in reproduction by schizophrenic parents. In L. C. Wynne, R. L. Cromwell & S. Matthysse (Eds.), *The nature of schizophrenia: New approaches to research and treatment* (pp. 401–29). New York: John Wiley and Sons.

Mednick, S. A. (1985). A learning theory approach to research in schizophrenia. *Psychological Bulletin*, **55**, 316–27.

Mednick, S. A. & Hefner, T. (1969). Reliability of developmental histories. *Pediatrics Digest*, **11**, 28–39.

Mednick, S. A., Machon, R. A., Huttunen, M. P. & Bonett, D. (1988). Adult schizophrenia following prenatal exposure to an influenza epidemic. *Archives of General Psychiatry*, **45**, 189–92.

Mednick, S. A., Mura, E., Schulsinger, F. & Mednick, B. (1971). Perinatal conditions and infant development in children with schizophrenic parents. *Social Biology*, **18** (suppl.), 103–33.

Mednick, S. A. & Schulsinger, F. (1965). A longitudinal study of children with a high risk for schizophrenia: A preliminary report. In S. Vandenberg (Ed.), *Methods and goals in human behaviour genetics* (pp. 255–96). New York: Academic Press.

Mednick, S. A. & Shaffer, J. (1963). Mother's retrospective reports in child rearing research. *American Journal of Orthopsychiatry*, **33**, 451–61.

Mednick, S. A. & Silverton, L. (1988). High-risk studies of the etiology of schizophrenia. In M. T. Tsuang & J. C. Simpson (Eds.), *Handbook of schizophrenia, vol. 3: Nosology, epidemiology and genetics*. Amsterdam: Elsevier.

Mirdal, G. K. M., Mednick, S. A., Schulsinger, F. & Fuchs, F. (1974). Perinatal complications in children of schizophrenic mothers. *Acta Psychiatrica Scandinavica*, **50**, 553–68.

Mura, E. L. (1974). Perinatal differences: a comparison of child psychiatric patients and their siblings. *Psychiatric Quarterly*, **48**, 239–55.

Murray, R. M., Reveley, A. M. & Lewis, S. W. (1988). Family history, obstetric complications and cerebral abnormality in schizophrenia. In M. T. Tsuang & J. C. Simpson (Eds.), *Handbook of schizophrenia, vol. 3: nosology, epidemiology, and genetics* (pp. 563–78). Amsterdam: Elsevier.

Nowakowski, R. S. (1987). Basic concepts of CNS development. *Child Development*, **58**, 568–95.

Parnas, J., Schulsinger, F., Teasdale, T. W., Schulsinger, H., Feldman, P. M. &

Mednick, S. A. (1982). Perinatal complications and clinical outcome within the schizophrenia spectrum. *British Journal of Psychiatry*, **140**, 416–20.

Pollack, M., Woerner, M. G., Goodman, W. & Greenberg, I. M. (1966). Childhood development patterns of hospitalized adult schizophrenic and nonschizophrenic patients and their siblings. *American Journal of Orthopsychiatry*, **36**, 510.

Pollin, W. & Stabenau, J. R. (1968). Biological, psychological and historical differences in a series of monozygotic twins discordant for schizophrenia. In D. Rosenthal & S. S. Kety (Eds.), *The Transmission of Schizophrenia*, pp. (317–32). London: Pergamon Press.

Reveley, A. M., Reveley, M. A. & Murray, R. M. (1984). Cerebral ventricular enlargement in non-genetic schizophrenia: A controlled twin study. *British Journal of Psychiatry*, **144**, 89–93.

Rieder, R. O., Bromans, S. H. & Rosenthal, D. (1977). The offspring of schizophrenics. II. Perinatal factors and IQ. *Archives of General Psychiatry*, **34**, 789.

Rutt, C. N. & Offord, D. R. (1971). Prenatal and perinatal complications in childhood schizophrenics and their siblings. *Journal of Nervous and Mental Disease*, **152**, 324–31.

Schulsinger, F., Parnas, J., Petersen, E. T., Schulsinger, H., Teasdale, T. W., Mednick, S. A., Moller, L. & Silverton, L. (1984). Cerebral ventricular size in the offspring of schizophrenic mothers. *Archives of General Psychiatry*, **41**, 602–6.

Schulsinger, H. (1976). A ten year follow-up of children of schizophrenic mothers: Clinical assessment. *Acta Psychiatrica Scandinavica*, **53**, 371–86.

Schwarzkopf, S. B., Nasrallah, H. A., Olson, S. C. & Coffman, J. A. (1989). Relationship of perinatal complications and genetic loading in schizohrenia. *Psychiatry Research*, **27**, 233–9.

Silverton, L., Finefellow, K. M., Mednick, S. A. & Schulsinger, F. (1985). Low birth weight and ventricular enlargement in a high-risk sample. *Journal of Abnormal Psychology*, **94**, 405–9.

Taft, L. T. & Goldfarb, W. (1964). Prenatal and perinatal factors in childhood schizophrenia. *Developmental Medicine and Child Neurology*, **6**, 32–43.

Terris, M., LaPouse, R. & Monk, M. A. (1964). The relation of prematurity and previous fetal loss to childhood schizophrenia. *American Journal of Psychiatry*, **121**, 476–81.

Torrey, E. F. & Hersch, S. P. (1975). Early childhood psychosis and bleeding during pregnancy: A prospective study of gravid women and their offspring. *Journal of Autism and Childhood Schizophrenia*, **5**(4), 287–97.

Torrey, E. F., Rawlings, R. & Waldman, P. (1988). Schizophrenic births and viral diseases in two states. *Schizophrenia Research*, **1**, 73–7.

Vorster, D. (1960). An investigation into the part played by organic factors in childhood schizophrenia. *Journal of Mental Science*, **106**, 494–522.

Wang, G. H. (1964). *Neural control of sweating*. Madison, Wisconsin: University of Wisconsin Press.

Whittam, H., Simon, G. B. & Mittler, P. J. (1966). The early development of psychotic children and their sibs. *Developmental Medicine and Child Neurology*, **8**, 552–60.

Woerner, M. G., Pollack, M. & Klein, D. F. (1971). Birth weight and length in schizophrenics, personality disorders, and their siblings. *British Journal of Psychiatry*, **118**, 461–4.

Woerner, M. G., Pollack, M. & Klein, D. F. (1973). Pregnancy and birth complications in psychiatric patients: A comparison of schizophrenic and personality disorder patients with their siblings. *Acta Psychiatrica Scandinavica*, **49**, 712–21.

Zitrin, A., Ferber, P. & Cohen, D. (1964). Pre- and perinatal factors in mental disorders of children. *Journal of Nervous and Mental Disease*, **121**, 357–61.

7

Possible interactions of obstetrical complications and abnormal fetal brain development in schizophrenia

MELVIN LYON AND CHRISTOPHER E. BARR

University of Southern California

Introduction

The purpose of this chapter is to describe briefly findings on brain pathologies in the early stages of fetal development. If a period of gestation (e.g. second trimester) is known to be disrupted in schizophrenia, this chronicle of developmental pathology might suggest which brain areas are likely to be affected. Conversely, if adult pathology studies of schizophrenic patients point to specific brain areas, then this chronicle may serve to delimit the period of gestation in which these areas develop most rapidly.

The following brief review selects those pathological features which are most commonly found, not specifically in schizophrenic populations, but in *unselected* comparison populations, such as that in the Collaborative Perinatal Project, sponsored by the National Institute of Neurological and Communicative Disorders and Stroke (Gilles, Leviton & Dooling, 1983; Freeman, 1985; Nelson & Ellenberg, 1986), with some additional emphasis on points which may be relevant to the etiology of schizophrenia. The Collaborative Perinatal Project study of neuropathology in fetal development is based on data from approximately 1100 brains of fetuses or infants representing a large sample of those who died during early development from an initial sample of more than 43000 pregnancies. These pathological data are therefore *unselected* in the sense that they relate only to those infants in the sample who died, mostly around the time of birth or shortly afterwards. Thus the evidence in surviving infants is meager, although some studies with brain imaging have been done. Nevertheless, attention has been paid to evidence found both in stillborn and liveborn infants and, where possible, these have been compared (see below).

Probably only about one-fifth of the causes known to be directly related to pathology of the brain can be shown to occur during the birth process itself, with the remaining four-fifths distributed over the time of pregnancy and development of the fetus. How these potential causes will actually affect brain growth is closely related to the stage of development at which the insult takes place. If the development of the fetal brain is divided into trimester periods, they may be characterized as follows with respect to growth activity and probable sources of pathology.

First trimester

During the initial development of the nervous system there is rapid growth of the brainstem and spinal cord. Within the developing ventricular space of the brain, the germinal mass, from which most of the telencephalic structures will develop, is a prominent structure. It can be divided into two general masses: the ganglionic mass, which will develop most prominently into the amygdala and caudato-putamen of the basal ganglia, and the extra-ganglionic mass from which the isocortex of the hemispheres will be a major development. Myelination is absent at this stage, and there is little evidence of glial activity related to myelination or repair of neural damage.

Genetic, infectional and nutritional factors can have general effects upon the structure and organization of brain and skull, and the brain does not produce hypertrophic astrocytes or macrophages in response to tissue insult. Any disturbances in brain growth at this stage will have far-reaching consequences, since the major cerebral and cerebellar structures remain to be developed, and severe malformations, or even death, may ensue.

Toward the end of the first trimester (see Fig. 7.1), there is a rapid acceleration in the growth of the germinal mass within the developing brain ventricles as the fetus begins to produce the major cerebral structures of the basal ganglia and much of the remaining telencephalon. This is the beginning of the great cell migration along radial fibers to the cortex and other structures (Rakic, 1988), which comes to dominate the second trimester (Gilles, Leviton & Dooling, 1983).

In summary, then, during the first trimester disturbances in development of the nervous system will show most frequently as retardation in general growth, since the differential growth spurt of specific hemispheric structures has not yet begun.

With respect to the CNS, the result may be a smaller cranium and brain size, yet sometimes without enlargement of the ventricles. Some studies of

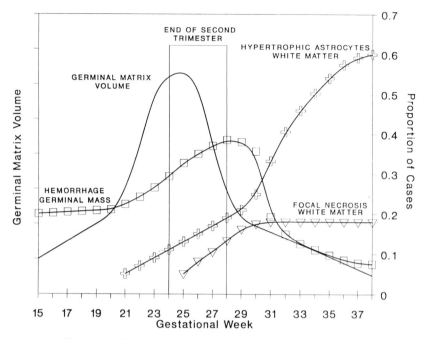

Figure 7.1. Timing of selected developmental and trauma-related processes during fetal neural development.

adult schizophrenic brains have found such a subgroup of individuals, and smaller brain-size measurements have been reported, especially for the frontal lobes (Andreasen *et al.*, 1986). When the smaller brain size is also accompanied by enlarged ventricles (perhaps as a result of perinatal complications, see below), these patients tend to have a negative schizophrenic symptomatology.

Second trimester

The second trimester is perhaps the most critical period in the development of the brain, since a large number of very rapid changes are taking place at once. In some cases, cells are migrating out from the germinal masses to form new structures, while in others, the original supporting structures for the earlier growth, which is now being completed, must be removed. For instance, when the major growth period of the basal ganglia is beginning to end, at the close of the second trimester, the germinal matrix within the ventricles disappears rather rapidly, and in the course of this dissolution it is

136

frequently the source of hemorrhages into the ventricular cavity or beneath the periventricular ependyma. Such intra- or periventricular hemorrhages are frequently found upon autopsy of prematurely-born infants, occurring just as frequently in live-born as in stillborn premature infants. This would seem to indicate that it is not birth trauma alone that causes this type of hemorrhage, but that factors preceding birth also play a role (Gilles, 1983c). Intraventricular hemorrhages, perhaps especially if they occur in conjunction with disruptions of the ependymal lining of the ventricles (Dooling, Chi & Gilles, 1983), may be accompanied by periventricular necrosis, which has been suggested as the possible cause of a corresponding enlargement of the lateral and third ventricles (Lancet, 1984). It may be relevant to note that Lesch & Bogerts (1984) have reported a reduction in thickness of the periventricular gray matter in schizophrenia.

Another major development during the second trimester is the laying out of the nuclear structure of the thalamus at about week 24, after which it begins a rapid enlargement, particularly of the dorsal thalamus, including the anterior nucleus, the dorsomedial nucleus, the geniculate bodies, and the pulvinar. The anterior nucleus is well-known for its wide limbic-system projection to the posterior cingulate gyrus; both this and its 'parallel' mesolimbic counterpart from ventral tegmentum to nucleus accumbens to medial and orbital prefrontal cortex, have been implicated in schizophrenia (Stevens, 1975).

Furthermore, the dorsomedial nucleus of the thalamus, which has a primary projection to the frontal pole of the neocortex, plays a major role in the striato-nigro-thalamo-cortical loop which may have much significance for dopaminergic systems. Dysfunction (Oke & Adams, 1987; Carlsson, 1989), or destruction (Pakkenberg & Gundersen, 1988), of this region have been related to brain development in schizophrenia.

The geniculates, pulvinar, and ventral posterolateral nucleus of the thalamus are especially important for the processing and integrating of sensory information from auditory, visual, and somesthetic sensory systems. It is also these regions, and their connections with sensory nuclei in the midbrain, which, according to evidence from studies of non-human primates, are among those most likely to be affected by birth complications, including asphyxia (Ranck & Windle, 1959; Faro & Windle, 1969).

Parallel with the thalamic development, the pallidal neurons are attaining full size, and the large cells of the striatum reach their full maturity by weeks 28–30 of gestation. The pattern of the principal sulci and gyri of the neocortex is also laid down during the second trimester, and by weeks 26–28 the layering of cells in the cerebral cortex is almost complete, with the line of Gennari appearing in the visual cortex. When cortical pathology appears, due to disturbance of the local blood supply, it is more likely to appear in the cortical 'border zones' which lie between the supplying branches of the middle and anterior cerebral arteries, or in the region lying between the distribution of the middle and posterior cerebral arteries. The regions principally affected are the frontal and parieto-temporal associational cortex, lying respectively rostral to the premotor area and caudal to the somatosensory cortex.

During the second trimester, the hippocampal formation is continuing its relatively stable progress and, in contrast to the isocortex and other structures, it reaches its final surface size in the beginning of the third trimester (Jammes & Gilles, 1983). From that point onward, the major developments lie in the synaptic connections and cellular arrangements within the structure. This process is exceptionally slow in CA1 as compared with CA2, and the dentate gyrus continues to increase its synaptic complement 2–4 months postnatally in the rhesus monkey (Rakic et al., 1986). As a consequence of this slow, relatively stable development, the hippocampal formation may still be subject to influences on cell migration and terminal connections long after other structures have achieved a relatively fixed structure. It is also thought that this very slow development of cells in some areas of the hippocampus has led to exaggerated accounts of cell atrophy and loss of fiber connections when brain samples are taken at, or around, the time of birth (Gilles, 1983a).

Along with the beginning of development of the cerebral cortex, the anterior vermis of the cerebellum reaches almost half of its folial development by the end of the second trimester. The second trimester also marks the start of the massive myelination of intracerebral axonal pathways, which is a process that is very sensitive to nutritional deficits, and which has great importance for effective brain function. The myelination process continues through the second and third trimesters, and in the case of the corticospinal tracts and certain cortical areas it may continue for the first years of life.

In terms of potential neuropathology, several features of growth during the second trimester deserve special notice. Discontinuities appear in the ependymal lining of the ventricles in three places, which potentially exposes these areas to greater danger from hydrostatic pressure changes in the ventricular fluid, such as might accompany hemorrhage or blocking of the ventricular foramina. These regions of most frequent ependymal disruption are in the occipital horns of the lateral ventricles, over the CA2 area of the hippocampus, and under the rostral corpus callosum. It is interesting to note, in light of the preceding observation, that these areas border on commonly-reported sites of neuropathology in the brains of schizophrenics (Andreasen et al., 1986; Bogerts, Meerts & Schonfeldt-Bausch, 1985; Jakob & Beckmann, 1986; Kovelman & Scheibel, 1984; McLardy, 1974). These regions continue

138

to be at greater risk of damage well up into the third trimester and beyond (see below).

With the growth of myelination, and the increasing visibility of fiber bundles within the brain, there can also be clear signs of leucoencephalopathy, usually as small infarcts, which are partial to the deep white matter of the frontal and parietal corpus callosum, typically some distance away from the periventricular wall. This necrosis is first detectable in the second trimester because, at this stage, microglia first appear in scar tissue, and hypertrophic astrocytes and macrophages also subsequently make their appearance.

The placement of these small lesions deep within the white matter may also be related to the distribution pattern of small blood vessels within these deeper regions (Leviton & Gilles, 1983). The significance of these findings for schizophrenic pathology is that the deep white matter involved frequently contains interhemispheric (callosal), and intracortical fiber tracts, both of which have frequently been implicated in schizophrenic dysfunction.

Because of the way in which the brain develops, with the hypothalamus and basal ganglia forming relatively early in the second trimester in the basal brain lateral to the sides of the third ventricle, and similarly due to the late-second-trimester dissolution of the germinal matrix, there is a greater chance that ventricular enlargement due to tissue loss may occur in the second trimester and that the earlier it occurs the more likely it will be that the third ventricle will also show enlargement.

Cortical atrophy alone, or together with lateral-ventricular enlargement but no third-ventricular enlargement, cannot as readily be associated with second-trimester development, since these changes are also known to occur as the result of perinatal ischemia. Even after the cellular migration to the cortex has largely been completed, the ependymal wall of the ventricles contains openings and weak spots resulting from the structural changes during rapid growth. At this time, increases in intraventricular pressure or hemorrhaging through the ventricular lining can more easily occur. However, it seems unlikely that these damage factors alone can be responsible for the ventriculomegaly commonly occurring in schizophrenia, since these two sources of damage are also found with high frequency in normally-developing children (Gilles, 1983b).

Some investigators have found evidence of periventricular gliosis, which is more likely to reflect previous injury or low-grade inflammation, possibly of viral etiology (e.g. Nieto & Escobar, 1972; Stevens, 1982). It should also be noted that evidence of gliosis would first become visible to the pathologist after damage during the second and third trimesters. On the other hand, cell loss in the periventricular regions is more likely to result from a necrotic process possibly related to, or reflected by, enlargement of the ventricular system. Although this enlargement could occur following second-trimester damage, it could also be due to perinatal trauma or to the interaction of (teratogenic or genetically-influenced) prenatal developmental disturbances with complications at delivery (see below).

Neurotransmitter systems

Besides the structural development during the second trimester, several important neurotransmitter systems begin to be evident. Of particular interest here are the dopaminergic (DA) and serotoninergic (5–HT) systems, both of which have been specifically implicated in schizophrenia (Carlsson, 1989; Sloviter, Damiano & Connor, 1980). These neurotransmitter systems appear to have their origins in the second trimester in the rat (Kalsbeek et al., 1988; Soinila et al., 1988). Dopaminergic cells are first detected on gestational days 13–14 in the rat fetus, a period roughly corresponding to the beginning of the second trimester in humans (Kalsbeek et al., 1988). The DA innervation of the mesencephalon and corpus striatum continues through the third trimester and the final innervation of prefrontal cortex DA connections is established after birth. In the rat, development of DA systems in the cortex continues until postnatal day 60, which roughly corresponds to early adulthood for these animals (Voorn et al., 1988).

In the mesencephalon, which would be the origin of the mesolimbic DA system suggested to be important in schizophrenia (Stevens, 1975; 1982), the DA cells separate into dorsal and ventral groups in the third trimester, and the primordial cells of the substantia nigra are visible just before birth (Voorn et al., 1988).

The available evidence on early development of 5–HT cells in the rat also indicates that this process begins during the second trimester in the peripheral nervous system (Soinila et al., 1988), with the development of noradrenergic cells occurring a few days later. Thus both DA and 5–HT systems are beginning to differentiate in a period corresponding to the second trimester, and both systems show a continuing development of fiber projections and innervation of cortical regions which proceeds postnatally as well.

Exposure to viral infection during the second trimester

The second trimester period has also been linked with the possible effects of viral infection in the mother upon the risk of schizophrenia developing in the child (Mednick *et al.*, 1988). This effect was *not* significant for the first- or third-trimester exposure to the same virus, which provides one of the few well-documented relationships of schizophrenia to a specific trimester period. Barr, Mednick & Munk-Jørgensen (1990) have surveyed the incidence of influenza and birthrate of schizophrenics in Denmark over a 40-year period. After removing the effect of season from the two variables, a significantly increased risk of schizophrenia was noted in those for whom months 6 or 7 of gestation fell in a period of higher influenza incidence.

Given that the viral infection is related to the later development of schizophrenia, how does it gain access to the brain? It has been difficult to demonstrate that the influenza virus itself survives for long in the maternal blood stream, let alone crosses the placental or fetal blood–brain barriers. However, Stagaard, Moos & Møllgård (see Chapter 5) have demonstrated the possibility that viral agents may, directly or indirectly, affect cellular development and migration in the fetal brain by receptor-mediated endocytosis. This would be most likely to occur in regions where the brain barrier systems had been weakened by processes such as those involved in the rapid proliferation and later removal by migration of the germinal masses around the ventricles (see above).

Conrad & Scheibel (1987) have theorized about a specific mechanism by which this might occur. They suggest that certain neuraminidase-bearing influenza viruses cross the fetal blood–brain barrier and disrupt neuronal migration. They propose that neuronal cell adhesion molecules (N-CAMs) control the migrational process by determining when the neuron adheres to the fiber it is following and when it disengages. They further hypothesize that the enzyme neuraminidase affects the adhesive characteristics of certain N-CAMs, so that when the neuraminidase-jacketed virus enters the fetal brain, neuronal migration may be interrupted.

Third trimester

At the beginning of the third trimester, the germinal matrix within the ventricles has largely disappeared and the neocortex is beginning its most extensive period of growth. The optic pathways become fully myelinated and the visual cortex develops rapidly during the third trimester (Kostovic & Rakic, 1984). The general plan of the sulci and gyri is now completed with the completion of the primary sulci and the appearance of the more varied secondary folds in the cortex. This process begins with prominent cellular migrations during months 4–6 of gestation, but the final synaptic development is not complete until well after birth. The synaptic development peaks with an overproduction of synapses postnatally, which later is reduced to the final adult number by a gradual process of attrition. The latter may, in fact, be the more essential process in the development of the finer cortical functions. In addition to these changes in synaptic number and configuration, the cerebral and cerebellar cortex show significant losses of superfluous neurons and retraction of axonal processes. This process continues throughout the third trimester and postnatally (Janowsky & Finlay, 1986). At about month 7, the development of the cerebellar cortex follows that of the neocortex, beginning with the migration of the granular cells from an overt position down to their final placement near the Purkinje cells. The anterior vermis develops before the lateral lobes of the cerebellum (Gilles *et al.*, 1983).

Third-trimester pathology related to schizophrenia

Some of the effects upon the fetus mentioned under the second trimester also apply to the third trimester. In particular, infection, hemorrhage and increased intraventricular pressure may result in brain tissue damage. In the third trimester, there should be clear residual evidence of gliosis for any substantial lesion.

The late development of the cerebellum, which results in some cells still being in mitotic stages at perinatal and even postnatal periods, means that this region is especially vulnerable to cell-loss in the third trimester. However, the region of the anterior vermis, which is evolutionarily an older part of the cerebellum, has been developing since the end of the second trimester, and it is therefore interesting to note that deficiencies in the foliation and size of the anterior vermis have also been detected in CT scans of schizophrenic brains (Heath, Franklin & Shraberg, 1979; Weinberger, Torrey & Wyatt, 1979; Cannon, Mednick & Parnas, 1989). These findings suggest that atrophy or dysgenesis has occurred specifically in the anterior cerebellar vermis of schizophrenic patients, and that the developmental disruption may have a second- or third-trimester origin.

Problems with eye movement coordination would also be related to damage involving the oldest part of the cerebellum, the flocculonodular lobe, which contains the most caudal part of the vermis, the nodule, or Xth vermal subdivision. This is also a region that would be most likely to sustain developmental damage during the late second, or early third, trimester (Gilles *et al.*, 1983).

It should also be noted that the cerebellar vermis appears to be essential for the long-term habituation of the startle response (Leaton & Supple, 1986), which is deficient in schizophrenics, and may have direct relevance to excessive autonomic nervous system responses in these patients (Swerdlow *et al.*, 1986).

Delivery

Birth traumas, or delivery complications, result most frequently in intraventricular, or subependymal, hemorrhage, with resultant damage most frequently within the white matter of the hemispheres. When the gray matter is affected directly, the sites most immediately at risk appear to be in the thalamus and upper brainstem. It has frequently been reported that perinatal hypoxia, or anoxia, may be directly related to brain damage, and that the hippocampus is especially sensitive to this effect (Hedner, 1978). Since the hippocampus has been implicated in both human (Mednick, 1970) and in animal (Schmajuk, 1987) theoretical models of schizophrenia, this possibility deserves attention. However, as far as can be determined from pathological samples taken from infants who died at or slightly before term, including some who must have suffered from perinatal hypoxia, the hippocampus and the basal ganglia, including the pallidum, rarely show clear pathological signs (Gilles, 1983b).

This does not rule out the possibility that perinatal anoxia can have less obvious effects. Hershkowitz, Grimm & Speiser (1983) found that postnatal (< 24 hours) anoxia, induced by breathing 100% nitrogen for 25 minutes in newborn rats, caused significant increases in the number of cholinergic muscarinic receptors in the hippocampus, which diminished after about 40 days, only to be replaced by a permanent increase in beta-adrenergic receptors in the same structure. The net weight of the hippocampi did not differ from that of control animals.

Enlargement of the cerebral ventricles may also occur, due to bleeding or to post-hemorrhagic hydrocephalus from blocked outflow of CSF. Ventricular dilatation is frequently associated with subependymal germinal matrix hemorrhage in very-low-birth-weight infants (Silverton et al., 1985). Such hemorrhages occur in about 40% of these infants, and a large number also show enlarged ventricles on CT scans. When the ventricles are enlarged, due to intraventricular hemorrhage or temporary hydrocephalus, it is usually associated with a loss of cellular substance from the thalamus and upper brainstem at the diencephalic–mesencephalic junction. Both the sensory nuclei of the tectum and the tegmentum of the midbrain, as well as the upper pons may be affected, and the cumulative effects would interfere especially with the integration and reception of sensory data (see also Ranck & Windle, 1959; Faro & Windle, 1969), as well as with the mesencephalic connections of the mesolimbic system which has been suggested to have special importance for many emotional and behavioral aspects of schizophrenia (Stevens & Livermore, 1978).

Birth complications have already been tied significantly to the abnormal

143

widening of the third ventricle in schizophrenics at age 33 (Schulsinger *et al.*, 1984; Silverton, *et al.*, 1985; Cannon *et al.*, 1989). With such enlargement of the ventricles, the third ventricle may also become enlarged and widened, taking on a 'barrel shape' rather than its normal narrow slit-like appearance in coronal sections. Hydrocephalus-induced pressure within the ventricles, even though it usually resolves spontaneously over time (Liechty *et al.*, 1983; Brann, 1985), almost certainly leads to a general loss of some periventricular cells, and there is reason to believe that this damage will be especially severe in those regions where the ependymal lining of the ventricles is interrupted. While the lining of the third ventricle is seldom directly broached in this manner, any connections between the hypothalamus and thalamus, or midbrain, will be in danger of disturbance. Likewise, the most common ependymal discontinuities within the ventricles, which may occur in all infants during development, lie close to the CA2 region of the hippocampus, the rostral and occipital parts of the corpus callosum, and the superior occipito-frontal bundle (Dooling *et al.*, 1983), so that these regions will all have a greater risk of damage when there is hemorrhagic bleeding and/or increased intraventricular pressure. There is also recent evidence from positron emission tomography studies that large hemorrhages, even in those infants that survive the insult without severe neurological signs, are accompanied by a marked impairment of blood flow in the white matter adjacent to the hemorrhagic area (Hill, Shackelford & Vollpe, 1984; Schub, Ahmann & Bain *et al.*, 1980).

Such deficits in neural functioning as would occur following these lesions, especially those involving the region at the diencephalic–mesencephalic border, could also result in the disruption of hypothalamic autonomic nervous system functions such as the excitatory hypothalamic control of sweating (Wang, 1964), loss of frontal and occipital interhemispheric cortical connections via the corpus callosum, and loss of coordination between the frontal and occipital cortical regions of the same side.

Pathological signs in the cortex are less frequent following birth trauma, but disturbances in the local blood supply to the cortex may show a greater tendency to cause damage in the so-called border-zones between the cerebral arterial fields, and these are found in the frontal and parietal associational cortex, as mentioned earlier. Extreme *hypo*tension, as a result of birth complications, may also be one of the potential causes of such damage, perhaps especially in view of the extremely fine diameter of many vessels in the terminal beds of the capillaries in the neonate.

It may also be added that when general stress factors affect the central nervous system of the fetus, pre- or perinatally, it is likely they do so with greater effect at the critical times and brain locations mentioned in this brief review.

Summary of delivery complications

Premature birth, which correlates highly with the known risk factor of low birth weight, drastically increases the risk of hypoxic episodes and of subependymal and intraventricular hemorrhage, which could result in necrosis and possibly in subsequent permanent enlargement of the ventricle. Periventricular structures are the most vulnerable to these complications, including particularly the gray matter of the thalamus, basal ganglia and hippocampus. It is also obvious that the hypothalamus and other limbic regions may be selectively damaged by enlargement to the third ventricle.

Third-ventricle enlargement appears to be involved in reduced autonomic nervous system activity, and this may provide a structural basis for some of the negative symptoms of schizophrenia (Cannon et al., 1988; Cannon, Mednick & Parnas, 1990). However, such direct periventricular damage may not be the only source of difficulty. In the brains of the unselected population of infants who died at or near the time of birth, there was far more frequently involvement of the deep white matter of the hemispheres than of obvious necrosis in gray matter (Gilles et al., 1983). This finding suggests that sudden changes in blood circulation, such as hypotension, or the presence of bacterial agents, drugs or endotoxins, may selectively attack the deeper white matter. The result may be that callosal and other interconnecting fiber bundles are defective, and that in postnatal development this results in further loss of cortical and subcortical cells and connections. It is suggestive for the interpretation of schizophrenic disturbances that such fiber-system losses are particularly frequent in the callosal interconnections of the frontal lobes, the superior occipito-frontal bundle, and the region of the callosum connecting the occipito-temporal association cortices.

Postnatal period

The period immediately following birth is especially complicated in premature delivery, and may be partly responsible for the known correlation between reduced birth weight (usually due to premature delivery) and later incidence of schizophrenia (Mednick & Silverton, 1988). Secondly, there are major features of cortical and cerebellar development that continue long after birth. These include the dendritic branching and synaptic proliferation of cortical cells, the 'programmed cell death' of cells resulting from initial overproduction (Rakic et al., 1986), and the repair of damage due to birth complications such as hemorrhage, etc.

Along with these general factors in growth and repair, it should be noted

145

that losses in subcortical cell structure may gradually be reflected in losses at the neocortical level due to the lack of appropriate subcortical afferent or efferent connections (Faro & Windle, 1969). This consideration is especially important with respect to the relationship between the basal ganglia, substantia nigra, dorsomedial thalamus and frontal cortex. Dysfunction of the subcortical connections within these interjoined structures may lead to reduced frontal cortex function (hypofrontality), which is one of the basic characteristics of adult schizophrenia (Carlsson, 1989).

Acknowledgements

This work was completed while Melvin Lyon was on leave of absence from Copenhagen University, Denmark, and was acting as Visiting Professor and Research Associate at the Social Sciences Research Institute, University of Southern California, Los Angeles, California, USA. Appreciation is expressed to SSRI director Ward Edwards and his colleagues and staff for providing facilities and encouragement in this work. Thanks are also expressed to William O. McClure, Floyd Gilles, Sarnoff Mednick and Tyrone Cannon for extremely useful discussions and comments. This research was also supported by a grant from the Scottish Rite Schizophrenia Researched Program and National Institute of Mental Health Grant 5R01 MH37692-04.

References

Andreasen, N., Nasrallah, H. A., Dunn, V., Olson, S. C., Grove, W. M., Erhardt, J. C., Coffman, J. A. & Crossett, J. H. W. (1986). Structural abnormalities in the frontal system in schizophrenia. *Archives of General Psychiatry*, **43**, 136–44.

Barr, C. E., Mednick, S. A. & Munk-Jørgensen, P. (1990). Exposure to influenza epidemics during gestation and adult schizophrenia: A 40 year study. *Archives of General Psychiatry*, **47**, 869–74.

Bogerts, B., Meertz, E. & Schonfeldt-Bausch, R. (1985). Basal ganglia and limbic system pathology in schizophrenia. *Archives of General Psychiatry*, **42**, 784–91.

Brann, A. W., Jr (1985). Factors during neonatal life that influence brain disorders. In J. M. Freeman (Ed.), *Prenatal and Perinatal Factors Associated with Brain Disorders* (pp. 263–358). National Institutes of Health Publication No. 85–1149. April 1985.

Cannon, T. D., Fuhrmann, M., Mednick, S. A., Machon, R. A., Parnas, J. & Schulsinger, F. (1988). Third ventricle enlargement and reduced electrodermal responsiveness. *Psychophysiology*, **25**, 153–6.

Cannon, T. D., Mednick, S. A. & Parnas, J. (1989). Genetic and perinatal determinants of structural brain deficits in schizophrenia. *Archives of General Psychiatry*, **46**, 883–9.

(1990). Antecedents of predominantly negative- and predominantly positive-symptom schizophrenia in a high-risk population. *Archives of General Psychiatry*, **47**, 622–32.

Carlsson, A. (1989). The current status of the dopamine hypothesis of schizophrenia. *Neuropsychopharmacology*, **1**(3), 179–86.

Conrad, A. J. & Scheibel, A. B. (1987). Schizophrenia and the hippocampus: The embryological hypothesis extended. *Schizophrenia Bulletin*, **13**(4), 577–87.

Dooling, E. C., Chi, J. G. & Gilles, F. H. (1983). Developmental changes in ventricular epithelia. In F. H. Gilles, A. Leviton & E. C. Dooling (Eds.), *The Developing Human Brain. Growth and Epidemiologic Neuropathology* (pp. 113–16). Boston: Wright PSG.

Faro, M. D. & Windle, W. F. (1969). Transneuronal degeneration in brains of monkeys asphyxiated at birth. *Experimental Neurology*, **24**, 38–53.

Freeman, J. M., (Ed.) (1985). *Prenatal and Perinatal Factors Associated with Brain Disorders*. National Institutes of Health Publication No. 85–1149. April, 1985.

Gilles, F. H. (1983a). Telencephalon medium and the olfacto-cerebral outpouching. In F. H. Gilles, A. Leviton & E. C. Dooling (Eds.), *The Developing Human Brain. Growth and Epidemiologic Neuropathology* (pp. 59–86). Boston: Wright PSG.

  (1983b). Neural damage: Inconstancy during gestation. In F. H. Gilles *et al.* (Eds.), *The Developing Human Brain. Growth and Epidemiologic Neuropathology* (pp. 227–43). Boston: Wright PSG.

  (1983c). Changes in growth and vulnerability at the end of the second trimester. In F. H. Gilles *et al.* (Eds.), *The Developing Human Brain. Growth and Epidemiological Neuropathology* (pp. 316–25). Boston: Wright PSG.

Gilles, F. H., Leviton, A. & Dooling, E. C. (1983). *The Developing Human Brain. Growth and Epidemiologic Neuropathology*. Boston: Wright PSG.

Heath, R. G., Franklin, D. E. & Shraberg, D. (1979). Gross pathology of the cerebellum in patients diagnosed and treated as functional psychiatric disorders. *Journal of Nervous and Mental Diseases*, **167**, 585–92.

Hedner, T. H. (1978). Central monoamine metabolism and neonatal oxygen deprivation. An experimental study in the rat brain. *Acta Physiologica Scandinavica, Suppl.* **460**, 1–34.

Hershkowitz, M., Grimm, V. E. & Speiser, Z. (1983). The effects of postnatal anoxia on behaviour and on the muscarinic and beta-adrenergic receptors in the hippocampus of the developing rat. *Developmental Brain Research*, **7**, 147–55.

Hill, A., Shackelford, G. & Vollpe, J. (1984). A potential mechanism of pathogenesis for early posthemorrhagic hydrocephalus in the premature newborn. *Pediatrics*, **73**, 19–21.

Jakob, H. & Beckmann, H. (1986). Prenatal developmental disturbances in the limbic allocortex in schizophrenia. *Journal of Neural Transmission*, **65**, 303–26.

Jammes, J. L. & Gilles, F. H. (1983). Telencephalic development: Matrix volume and isocortex and allocortex surface areas. In F. H. Gilles, A. Leviton & E. C. Dooling (Eds.), *The Developing Human Brain. Growth and Epidemiologic Neuropathology* (pp. 87–93). Boston: Wright PSG.

147

Janowsky, J. S. & Finlay, B. L. (1986). The outcome of perinatal brain damage: The role of normal neuron loss and axon retraction. *Developmental Medicine and Child Neurology*, **26**, 375–89.

Kalsbeek, A., Voorn, P., Buijs, R. M., Pool, C. W. & Uylings, H. B. (1988). Development of the dopaminergic innervation in the prefrontal cortex of the rat. *Journal of Comparative Neurology*, **269**(1), 58–72.

Kostovic, I. & Rakic, P. (1984). Development of prestriate visual projections in the monkey and human fetal cerebrum revealed by transient cholinesterase staining. *The Journal of Neuroscience*, **4**, 25–42.

Kovelman, J. A. & Scheibel, A. B. (1984). A neurohistological correlate of schizophrenia. *Biological Psychiatry*, **19**, 1601–21.

Lancet, The (1984). Ischaemia and haemorrhage in the premature brain. Editorial of October 13, 1984.

Leaton, R. L. & Supple, W. F., Jr (1986). Cerebellar vermis: Essential for long-term habituation of the acoustic startle response. *Science*, **232**, 513–15.

Lesch, A. & Bogerts, B. (1984). The diencephalon in schizophrenia: Evidence for reduced thickness of the periventricular gray matter. *European Archives of Psychiatry and Neurological Science*, **234**, 212–19.

Leviton, A. & Gilles, F. H. (1983). Etiologic relationships among the perinatal telencephalic leucoencephalopathies. In F. H. Gilles *et al.* (Eds.), *The Developing Human Brain. Growth and Epidemiologic Neuropathology* (pp. 304–15). Boston: Wright PSG.

Liechty, E. A., Gilmor, R. L., Bryson, C. Q. & Bull, M. J. (1983). Outcome of high-risk neonates with ventriculomegaly. *Developmental Medicine and Child Neurology*, **25**, 162–8.

McLardy, T. (1974). Hippocampal zinc and structural deficit in brains from chronic alcoholics and some schizophrenics. *Journal of Orthomolecular Psychiatry*, **4**(1), 32–6.

Mednick, S. A. (1970). Breakdown in individuals at high risk for schizophrenia: possible predispositional perinatal factors. *Mental Hygiene*, **54**(1), 50–63.

Mednick, S. A., Machon, R. A., Huttunen, M. O. & Bonnett, D. (1988). Adult schizophrenia following prenatal exposure to an influenza epidemic. *Archives of General Psychiatry*, **45**, 189–92.

Mednick, S. A. & Silverton, L. (1988). High-risk studies of the etiology of schizophrenia. In M. T. Tsuang & J. C. Simpson (Eds.), *Handbook of Schizophrenia, Vol. 3: Nosology, Epidemiology and Genetics* (pp. 543–62). Amsterdam: Elsevier.

Nelson, K. B. & Ellenberg, J. H. (1986). Antecedents of cerebral palsy. Multivariate analysis of risk. *New England Journal of Medicine*, **315**, 81–6.

Nieto, D. & Escobar, A. (1972). Major psychoses. In J. Minkler (Ed.), *Pathology of the Nervous System* (pp. 2654–65). New York: McGraw-Hill.

Oke, A. F. & Adams, R. N. (1987). Elevated thalamic dopamine: Possible link to sensory dysfunctions in schizophrenia. *Schizophrenia Bulletin*, **13**, 589–603.

Pakkenberg, B. & Gundersen, H. J. G. (1988). Total number of neurons and glial cells in human brain nuclei estimated by the dissector and the fractionator. *Journal of Microscopy*, **150**, 1–20.

Rakic, P. (1988). Defects of neuronal migration and the pathogenesis of cortical

148

malformations. In G. J. Boer, M. G. P. Feenstra, M. Mirmiran, D. F. Swaab & F. van Haaren (Eds.), *Progress in Brain Research* (Vol. 73, pp. 15–37). Amsterdam: Elsevier.

Rakic, P., Bourgeois, J-P., Eckenhoff, M. F., Zecevic, N. & Goldman-Rakic, P. S. (1986). Concurrent overproduction of synapses in diverse regions of the primate cerebral cortex. *Science*, **232**, 232–5.

Ranck, J. B., Jr & Windle, W. F. (1959). Brain damage in the monkey, *Macaca mulatta*, by asphyxia neonatorum. *Experimental Neurology*, **1**, 130–54.

Schmajuk, N. A. (1987). Animal models for schizophrenia: The hippocampally lesioned animal. *Schizophrenia Bulletin*, **13**(2), 317–27.

Schub, H. S., Ahmann, P. & Bain, R., et al. (1980). Long-term developmental follow-up of premature infants with subependymal intraventricular hemorrhage: Reason for optimism. *Clinical Research*, **28**, 874A.

Schulsinger, F., Parnas, J., Petersen, E. T., Schulsinger, H., Teasdale, T. W., Mednick, S. A., Moller, L. & Silverton, L. (1984). Cerebral ventricular size in the offspring of schizophrenic mothers. *Archives of General Psychiatry*, **41**, 602–6.

Silverton, L., Finello, K. M., Mednick, S. A., Schulsinger, F. & Parnas, J. (1985). Birthweight, schizophrenia and ventricular enlargement in a high risk sample. *Journal of Abnormal Psychology*, **94**, 405–9.

Sloviter, R. S., Damiano, B. P. & Connor, J. D. (1980). Relative potency of amphetamine isomers in causing the serotonin behavioral syndrome in rats. *Biological Psychiatry*, **15**, 789–96.

Soinila, S., Ahonen, M., Joh, T. H. & Steinbusch, H. W. (1988). 5–Hydroxytryptamine and catecholamines in developing sympathetic cells of the rat. *Journal of the Autonomic Nervous System*, **22**(3), 193–202.

Stevens, J. R. (1975). GABA blockade, dopamine and schizophrenia: Experimental activation of the mesolimbic system. *International Journal of Neurology*, **10**, 115–27.

Stevens, J. R. (1982). Neuropathology of schizophrenia. *Archives of General Psychiatry*, **39**, 1131–9.

Stevens, J. R. & Livermore, A., Jr (1978). Kindling of the mesolimbic dopamine system: Animal model of psychosis. *Neurology*, **28**, 36–46.

Swerdlow, N. R., Braff, D. L., Geyer, M. A. & Koob, G. F. (1986). Central dopamine hyperactivity in rats mimics abnormal acoustic startle response in schizophrenics. *Biological Psychiatry*, **21**, 23–33.

Voorn, P., Kalsbeek, A., Jorritsma-Byham, B. & Groenewegen, H. J. (1988). The pre- and postnatal development of the dopaminergic cell groups in the ventral mesencephalon and the dopaminergic innervation of the striatum of the rat. *Neuroscience*, **25**(3), 857–87.

Wang, G. H. (1964). *The Neural Control of Sweating*. Madison: University of Wisconsin Press.

Weinberger, D. R., Torrey, E. F. & Wyatt, R. J. (1979). Cerebellar atrophy in chronic schizophrenia. *Lancet I*, 718–19.

Part V

Neuropathological abnormalities in schizophrenia

8

The neuropathology of schizophrenia: pathophysiological and neurodevelopmental implications

BERNHARD BOGERTS

University of Düsseldorf

Introduction

There is probably no other neuropsychiatric disease that is more challenging to neuroanatomists and neuropathologists than schizophrenia. After the classical era of neuromorphological schizophrenia research failed to demonstrate convincingly structural alterations in brains of schizophrenics, this disease became a battlefield of different psychiatric world conceptions and ideologies. However, these generally suffered from the same flaws as the early neuropathological studies did; namely, the lack of replicable empirical data derived from well-controlled quantitative–statistical studies.

Another reason which led many psychiatrists, psychologists and neuroscientists to the assumption that schizophrenia is a disease of the mind rather than a disease of the brain was that, until recently, little was known about the neuroanatomy and physiology of the brain systems involved in functions that are now thought to be disturbed in schizophrenia. Such brain functions comprise the coordination of cognitive and emotional activities, the higher cortical integration and association of different sensory modalities, sensory gating, and the neuronal generation and control of basic drives and emotions. The increasing knowledge in these fields of neuroscience and a considerable number of brain imaging and post-mortem brain studies give evidence that abnormal brain morphology and physiology are essential biological components of the disease and provide compelling arguments against concepts that argue that the disease is mainly a result of psychosocial influences.

A new era of neuromorphological schizophrenia research, receiving strong impetus from the introduction of neuroimaging techniques such as computed tomography (CT) and magnetic resonance imaging (MRI), started in the early 1970s. Contrary to investigations in the first half of the century, many of the new studies applied quantitative statistical methods and investigated brain regions, the physiology of which became known in the last two decades and which are now regarded to be crucial for the pathophysiology of the disease. The majority of the more recent post-mortem studies agree that there is limbic pathology in schizophrenia and that the anatomical anomalies reflect a disorder of early brain development.

There are several excellent reviews on the earlier neuromorphological studies in schizophrenia (David, 1957; Peters, 1967; Nieto & Escobar, 1972; Weinberger, Wagner & Wyatt, 1983; Kirch & Weinberger, 1986; Stevens, 1982; Kovelman & Scheibel, 1986; Roberts & Crow, 1987). The present article will focus on the more recent qualitative and quantitative studies published since 1970, and addresses the following questions:

(1) What neuromorphological alterations have been described and which clues to the etiology do they give?
(2) How strong is the empirical evidence for these findings?
(3) Can some symptoms of schizophrenia be explained by the reported brain anomalies?
(4) How can abnormal brain morphology be related to the typical course of the disease?

What neuromorphological alterations have been described and which clues to the etiology do they give?

Since 1970, more than 30 post-mortem brain studies on schizophrenia have been published. The reports can be subdivided into: (1) those that are consistent with a disorder of brain development; (2) those that favor an inflammatory or degenerative brain disease; and (3) those that do not comment on the etiology of the reported anomalies.

Findings consistent with a disorder of brain development

McLardy (1974) reported that 12 out of 30 brains from early-onset schizophrenics (compared to seven controls) had a bilateral strikingly-abnormal granule cell layer in the dentate gyrus of the hippocampal formation. The depth of the layer was reduced from its normal range of 7–5 nerve cell bodies to about 4 cell bodies. Under higher light-microscope powers, individual granule cells appeared normal in cytoplasm and nucleus.

Zinc content of the granule cell layer was reduced by 50%. McLardy concluded that the cell picture was not suggestive of a degenerative appearance, but rather was consistent with a developmental arrest. He further suggested that in about one-third of schizophrenics, a genetic factor, or a perinatal environmental factor, or a combination of both, had prevented granule cells from mitoting to their normal numerosity. Regions other than hippocampal granule cell layer were not investigated in this study.

To find out whether ventricular enlargement, as revealed by neuroradio-logical methods, is caused by a regionally localizable or by a more diffuse lack of brain tissue, we performed volume measurements of several parts of the basal ganglia and limbic system using myelin-stained serial sections of left hemispheres of 13 schizophrenics (10 controls) belonging to the Vogt collection (Bogerts, 1984; Bogerts et al., 1985). All patients died before the introduction of neuroleptic drugs, and none had been treated with insulin or electroconvulsive therapy. The schizophrenics displayed, on the average, a significant volume-reduction of the limbic parts of the temporal lobe (amygdala, hippocampus, parahippocampal gyrus), by 20–30%. The volume of the internal pallidum was 20% smaller, while the volumes of the external pallidum, caudate nucleus, putamen and nucleus accumbens were unchanged. According to the concept of pathoclisis introduced by Vogt (1925), we concluded that the internal pallidum and limbic temporal lobe structures could be selectively vulnerable to various noxious agents, such as viruses, toxic substances and perinatal hypoxia, or that an inherited congenital hypoplasia of these structures might form a predisposition to the disease.

Kovelman & Scheibel (1984) performed, in 10 chronic schizophrenic patients (8 controls), measurements of pyramidal-cell orientation in all CA-segments of the hippocampal formation. An apparently consistent alteration of pyramidal cell orientation was found, particularly in anterior and middle hippocampal regions. Cell disarray was most pronounced at the CA1/prosubiculum and CA1/CA2 interfaces. In this study, qualitative findings reported in a previous paper by the same group (Scheibel & Kovelman, 1981) were confirmed. The structural alterations were considered suggestive of defective patterns of neuronal migration during embryological development of the brain. Similar measurements of hippocampal pyramidal-cell orientation were repeated by Altshuler et al. (1987) in a group of seven schizophrenics (6 controls) of the Yakovlev collection. Though statistical analysis failed to reveal significantly greater pyramidal-cell disorganization in the schizophrenics, the data suggested a relationship between the degree of pyramidal-cell disarray and the severity of behavioral impairment due to psychosis.

Quantitative morphometric determinations of neuronal and glial density, neuron–glia ratios and neuronal size were performed by Benes, Davidson & Bird (1986) in the prefrontal, anterior cingulate, and primary motor cortex of 10 schizophrenics (10 controls). The neuronal density was significantly lower in layer VI of the prefrontal cortex, layer V of the cingulate gyrus, and layer III of the motor cortex. An additional analysis of the arrangement of neurons in the anterior cingulate gyrus, which is a part of the limbic system, revealed that aggregates of neurons are smaller in size and separated by wider distances than those observed in the controls (Benes, 1987). The number of glia per unit volume was generally lower in the schizophrenics. The data argued compellingly against the occurrence of a progressive neuronal degeneration; the possibility was suggested that a nondegenerative cytoarchitectural variation, caused by a neuronal dropout early in life, might be present in the schizophrenic cingulate cortex.

Jakob & Beckmann (1986) examined 64 autopsied brains of schizophrenics (as controls, 7 oligophrenics, 2 patients with organic syndrome, and 1 with personality disorder were used). Forty-two schizophrenics were reported to have an abnormally developed temporal lobe with an unusual pattern of temporal sulci and gyri. Twenty of these 42 cases had cytoarchitectonic abnormalities in the rostral entorhinal region of the parahippocampal gyrus, mainly a poorly-developed structure in the upper layers with heterotopic displacement of single pre-alpha cell groups. Sixteen cases revealed an abnormal structure of the ventral insular cortex. Other brain regions were not investigated; gliosis could not be observed. The reported changes were based on qualitative brain-tissue assessment and did not have morphometric–statistical backing. The finding suggested a disturbance of neuronal migration in the allocortex during the second trimester of pregnancy.

Further morphometric examinations on all segments of the hippocampal formation (Falkai & Bogerts, 1986) and of the entorhinal region (Falkai, Bogerts & Rozumek, 1988a) of 13 schizophrenics (11 controls) were performed in the Vogt collection. The volumes of the hippocampal segments CA1/CA2, CA3, CA4 and dentate gyrus were reduced, whereas no significant volume reduction of the alveus, fimbria hippocampi and subicular region could be found. The perforant path showed a trend towards volume reduction. The absolute number of nerve cells was reduced in CA1/CA2, CA3, CA4 and in the granule cell layer of the dentate gyrus by 10–30%, whereas the mean absolute number and density of glial cells did not differ between patients and controls. Comparable significant reductions in structure, volume and nerve-cell numbers without increased glial-cell numbers were obtained for the entorhinal cortex of the same patients. The absence of gliosis in hippocampus and entorhinal cortex and obvious shape alterations of the hippocampal formation of some schizophrenics (Bogerts, 1989), which could hardly be explained by pathological influences occurring later in life such as atrophic processes or viral infections, were taken as indicative of a developmental disturbance occurring very early in childhood and argued against an ongoing progressive brain disease.

In order to investigate quantitatively whether there is an unusual location of pre-alpha cell clusters in deeper layers of the entorhinal cortex of schizophrenics indicating disturbances of neuronal migration of these entorhinal cell groups during fetal development, as suggested by Jakob & Beckmann (1986), we measured in 7 schizophrenics (11 controls) of the Vogt collection and 11 recently-collected brains of schizophrenics (plus 11 new controls) the distance between the pial surface of the entorhinal cortex and the center of pre-alpha cell clusters, and calculated the ratio of this parameter to the thickness of the whole entorhinal cortex (Falkai et al., 1988b). Four of the schizophrenics of the Vogt collection and 3 of the recently-collected brains of schizophrenics had values above control range, indicating a disturbance of pre-alpha cell migration from the inner to the outer layers of the entorhinal cortex during fetal development in these cases. Group means for distances between entorhinal cortical surface and pre-alpha cell clusters differed significantly by about 30% for the brains of the Vogt collection and showed a trend towards increased values (by 20%) for the brains of our new collection.

Recently, Altshuler et al. (1988) measured hippocampal and para-hippocampal gyrus cross-sectional areas at the level of the mamillary body in 12 schizophrenics. The parahippocampal cortex was significantly smaller in the schizophrenics, as compared with 10 normal controls but not to 17 suicide patients. Furthermore, there was a significant shape distortion of hippocampus and parahippocampal cortex in the schizophrenics.

Reports consistent with an inflammatory or degenerative brain disease

Nieto & Escobar (1972), using silver–lithium carbonate staining for glial fibrils, investigated brains of 10 schizophrenics (4 controls) and described, by qualitative tissue assessment, gliosis in various brainstem structures surrounding the third ventricle and aqueduct; gliosis in the hippocampus was found in 4 of the 10 patients.

Fisman (1975) examined qualitatively the brainstem (medulla, pons, midbrain) of 24 psychiatric patients, 10 of them suffering from paranoid–hallucinatory psychosis (10 controls). Glial knots and perivascular infiltrations, interpreted as encephalitic in origin, were found in 7 out of the 10 paranoid–hallucinatory patients.

The nucleus of the ansa lenticularis, a part of the basal nucleus, was studied by Averback (1981). Cellular degeneration and cytoplasmatic vacuolation resembling the so-called 'dwarf cells' described by the Vogts fifty years ago, were found in 11 of 13 schizophrenics (35 controls). No morphometric methods were used.

Stevens (1982) investigated histologic brain sections of 25 schizophrenic patients and compared them qualitatively with similarly-prepared sections from the same brain regions of 28 non-schizophrenic psychiatric patients and 20 age-matched non-psychiatric patients. Holzer's stain for glial fibrils demonstrated: 16 schizophrenic cases had periventricular hypothalamic gliosis; 9–12 schizophrenics had gliosis in midbrain tegmentum, bed nucleus of the stria terminalis, basal nucleus, medial thalamus, amygdala and hippocampus; 9 cases had neuron loss or abnormal mineralization in the pallidum, and 13–15 cases had ependymal granulations or corpora amylacea. Stevens felt that the nature and distribution of the findings suggested previous or low-grade inflammation, possibly due to a virus.

Nasrallah et al. (1983) investigated histologically the corpus callosum of 11 early-onset and seven late-onset schizophrenics and seven manic-depressive patients (11 medical or surgical control cases). The number of glial nuclei (hematoxylin–eosin stain) and collosal fibers (Bielschowsky stain) was counted in randomly preselected squares on a grid. No differences in glial-cell densities and callosal-fiber densities between schizophrenics, manic-depressives and controls were found. Blind gliosis rating by a neuropathologist, however, revealed significantly more gliosis in late-onset schizophrenia compared to early-onset schizophrenia (anteriorly and posteriorly) and controls (anteriorly). In two previous studies, the same group found a strong trend ($p = 0.08$) for the early-onset schizophrenic subgroup to have a thicker corpus callosum than the late-onset schizophrenic subgroup (Nasrallah et al., 1979). In a re-analysis of the measurements, the difference between early- and late-onset schizophrenia, as well as the difference between early-onset schizophrenia and controls, was significant only for the frontal but not for the posterior part of the corpus callosum (Bigelow, Nasrallah & Rauscher, 1983).

Studies with no comments on etiology

In a study of post-mortem brain volume measurements, Rosenthal & Bigelow (1972) found in a group of 10 schizophrenics (10 controls) an insignificant increase in total cortical volume, thalamic volume, and temporal lobe volume; the average corpus callosum width stood out as being significantly increased. This study was criticized because: (1) volumes were determined by using very thick sections (about 1 cm); (2) a number of controls suffered from personality disorders or from chronic alcoholism, which is known to cause brain atrophy; (3) by contrast with these results, the vast majority of CT studies demonstrated a moderate brain atrophy in many schizophrenics.

Dom *et al.* (1981) performed cell-density and cell-size studies of inter-neurons in the nucleus accumbens, caudate, putamen and thalamus anterior, medialis, lateralis and posterior, of five catatonic schizophrenics (five controls) from the Vogt collection. In striatum and accumbens, no significant differences in cell densities were found although a slight decrease in size of Golgi Type II neurons was described. In the posterior thalamus of the schizophrenics, microneuron density was reduced by 40%.

In our first morphometric study (Bogerts, Häntsch & Herzer, 1983a) we evaluated in the Vogt collection the lateral (nigrostriatal) and medial (mesolimbic) parts of the mesencephalic dopaminergic systems of six schizophrenics (six controls). There was a significant volume reduction, by about 21%, of the lateral parts of the substantia nigra, and the size of the nerve-cell bodies was significantly reduced in the medial part by 16%. The number of neurons was unaltered in both the mesolimbic and nigrostriatal segment. The findings in the lateral part of the substantia nigra suggested a reduction of neuropil consisting of afferent fibers from striatum and cortex; the reduced cell size of the medial, mesolimbic, neurons was taken as indicative of a dopaminergic underactivity rather than overactivity of these cells in the schizophrenics investigated.

Volume measurements and linear measurements of the whole thalamus and of all large thalamic subnuclei (nuclei anterior, medialis, lateralis, reticularis, dorsalis superficialis, central cell group, pulvinar, medial and lateral geniculate body, periventricular gray matter) of 15 schizophrenics of the Vogt collection (12 controls) were performed by Lesch and Bogerts (1984). No volume differences in any of these thalamic structures could be detected, with the exception of the central thalamic cell group, which showed a trend towards smaller volumes (by 20%) in the schizophrenics, and of the thickness of the periventricular gray matter, which was significantly reduced by some 20%.

Brown *et al.* (1986) studied 41 schizophrenic patients (controls were 29 patients with affective disorder) of the Runwell collection, UK. On photographs of one section of each brain, the area of several parts of the cortex, basal ganglia, limbic system and ventricles was measured planimetri-cally. The schizophrenics' brains were 6% lighter (equivalent to some 50 grams of brain tissue), and the lateral ventricles were larger in the anterior (by 19%) and temporal (by 97%) horn cross-sectional areas. The para-hippocampal gyrus was 11% thinner; hippocampus and amygdala were not measured. The findings provided post-mortem confirmation that ventricular enlargement in schizophrenia is particularly associated with loss of limbic brain tissue surrounding the temporal horn such as hippocampus and amygdala. The same group (Colter *et al.*, 1987) reported a reduction of the white matter of the parahippocampal gyrus (by 23%) in a sample of 17 patients (11 affective controls).

Jeste & Lohr (1989) determined volumes and pyramidal cell densities in each of the four CA-sectors of the cornu ammonis in the right and left anterior hippocampi from 13 schizophrenic patients (9 leucotomized and 16 normal controls) of the Yakovlev collection. Sections from schizophrenic patients had almost consistently the lowest volume and pyramidal cell density in all sectors. The differences were greatest in left CA4 with schizophrenic patients having significantly lower pyramidal cell density than normal controls and significantly lower volume than leucotomy controls.

Pakkenberg (1987) investigated 6-mm-thick whole-brain serial sections of 29 chronic schizophrenic patients (30 controls). The volumes of both hemispheres, of the cortex and subcortical white matter and the brain weight (by 110 grams) were significantly reduced, whereas ventricular volume was increased. Type II patients (according to Crow) had significantly larger ventricles than Type I schizophrenics.

Lohr & Jeste (1988) undertook volume measurements and cell counts in the noradrenergic locus ceruleus of 15 schizophrenics of the Yakovlev collection. There was a trend for decreased locus ceruleus volume without loss of neurons, indicating a reduction of neuropil in the schizophrenics as compared with leucotomized controls. The results appeared comparable to those described in the substantia nigra (Bogerts *et al.*, 1983a).

Investigations on glial cells

Whether or not there is gliosis in brains of schizophrenics is still a controversial issue. If the reported structural anomalies reflect developmental disturbances, perinatal complications or inherited variations, one would not expect gliosis, since only pathological events occurring after birth, e.g. atrophic processes or viral infections, are associated with increased glial-cell densities (Oyanagi, Yoshida & Icuta, 1986; Larroche, 1984). The immature brain is not capable of reactive gliosis.

Two qualitative studies reported gliosis in the amygdala and the hippocampus in 4 out of 10 (Nieto & Escobar, 1972) and 9 out of 28 schizophrenics (Stevens, 1982). One qualitative study found no gliosis in the medial temporal lobe of schizophrenics (Jakob & Beckmann, 1986). The major problem with these qualitative studies of gliosis is that they do not allow a quantitative–statistical comparison of glial cell densities. In six controlled quantitative studies (Falkai & Bogerts, 1986; Falkai *et al.*, 1988a; Benes, 1987; Roberts *et al.*, 1986; 1987; Stevens *et al.*, 1988), no evidence of gliosis in the medial temporal lobe, cingulate gyrus or hypothalamic periventricular regions could be found. It has been argued that in some of these studies the applied densitometric methods for assessing glial fibrillary acidic protein levels were not sensitive enough to detect moderate degrees of gliosis (Casanova, Stevens & Bigelow, 1987; Stevens *et al.*, 1988). Moreover, all of these studies investigated relatively small samples in which a moderate gliosis, if any, in a subgroup of patients, would not have been detected by the applied statistical tests. But at the same time in the above-mentioned qualitative studies, the majority of schizophrenics do not exhibit gliosis in the medial temporal lobe. Likewise, we could not detect increased glial-cell densities even in the smallest hippocampi of schizophrenics of the Vogt collection.

If corroborated by future studies with large sample sizes, the lack of gliosis in hypo- or dysplastic brain areas of schizophrenics would strongly support the notion that the structural deviations are either already present at birth or acquired as a result of perinatal complications, which can cause only transient gliosis. Alternatively, they could reflect a failure of the hippocampus to develop completely during the first year of life due to a deficiency of adequate environmental stimuli (Greenough & Zuraske, 1979; Walsh, 1981).

How strong is the empirical evidence for the recent neuroanatomical findings?

Nearly all studies performed since 1970 revealed that the brain anomalies detected in schizophrenics are subtle and not comparable in extent to the changes seen in degenerative brain diseases such as Alzheimer's, Parkinson's and Huntington's disease. Another important difference from these diseases is that, for the affected brain regions, the values from schizophrenics considerably overlap the range of controls.

With respect to the considerable variability of normal brain structure, more subtle abnormalities of macroscopic and microscopic brain anatomy can only be evidenced by applying adequate quantitative–statistical proce- dures; these were not available during the first half of the century when most neuropathological studies on schizophrenia had been published, and have not been applied by some of the above-mentioned studies.

Qualitative brain-tissue assessment as used in the studies summarized in Table 8.1 are very useful in describing well-known and obvious histological changes as seen in vascular, traumatic, infectious and degenerative brain diseases. The application of such methods is problematic in defining more subtle alterations in brain histology. To demonstrate such changes convin- cingly, quantitative–statistical evidence for group differences is necessary

Table 8.1. *Qualitative post-mortem studies of limbic structures in schizophrenia*

Study	Findings
Nieto & Escobar (1972)	Gliosis in the hippocampus, 4 of 10 patients
McLardy (1974)	Reduced thickness of the granule cell layer in the hippocampal formation
Averback (1981)	Cellular degeneration in the nucleus of the ansa lenticularis
Stevens (1982)	Gliosis in the hippocampus and amygdala in 6 of 25 patients
Jakob & Beckmann (1986)	Cytoarchitectonic abnormalities in the rostral entorhinal region, abnormal pattern of temporal sulci

when taking into account the considerable anatomical variation of normal and and abnormal structures. During the first half of the century the controversies characteristic for neuropathology of schizophrenia were mainly caused by the methodological flaws associated with only qualitative brain tissue assessment.

At the present time, most psychiatrists agree that schizophrenia may comprise a group of disorders rather than a single disease entity; hence, no uniform or 'specific' morphological alterations can be expected. The clinical inhomogeneity and the enormous variation of the normal and pathological brain anatomy require relatively large and well-matched samples of patients and controls. Furthermore, we feel that, for quantitative evaluation, serial brain sections are necessary to insure comparisons of identical anatomical levels and to make it possible to assess the whole anterio-posterior, medio-lateral and cranio-caudal extent of the structure in question.

Until recently, there was no brain collection that fulfilled all of these requirements. Most of the recent morphometric studies investigated material of the Vogt collection in Düsseldorf, Germany, the Yakovlev collection in Washington DC, USA, or the Runwell collection in Wickford, Essex, UK. In the Vogt and Yakovlev collections, serial sections of whole brains or hemispheres of only 10–15 brains of schizophrenics (most of them were never treated with neuroleptic drugs or electroconvulsive therapy) are available for quantitative evaluation. All schizophrenics in the Yakovlev collection were leucotomized; therefore, other leucotomized cases (intractable pain patients) of the collection were used as controls. This is problematic because of the variable extent and site of leucotomies. In the Vogt collection, schizophrenics and controls are poorly sex-matched, some midline structures such as septum

Table 8.2. *Morphometric post-mortem studies of limbic structures in schizophrenia*

Study	Findings
Bogerts (1984)	Reduced volumes of hippocampus, parahip-
Bogerts *et al.* (1985)	pocampal gyrus and amygdala
Kovelman & Scheibel (1984)	Disarray of hippocampal pyramidal cells
Lesch & Bogerts (1984)	Reduced thickness of diencephalic periven-
	tricular gray matter
Brown *et al.* (1986)	Reduced thickness of parahippocampal cortex;
	temporal horn enlargement
Falkai & Bogerts (1986)	Reduction of hippocampal pyramidal cells
Benes *et al.* (1986)	Lower neuronal densities and cytoarchitec-
Benes (1987)	tural disturbances in the cingulate gyrus
Colter *et al.* (1987)	Reduced parahippocampal white matter
Altshuler *et al.* (1987)	Correlation between hippocampal pyramidal
	cell disarray and severity of clinical symptoms
Falkai *et al.* (1988a)	Lower volume and cell densities in the ento-
	rhinal cortex
Falkai *et al.* (1988b)	Abnormal location of entorhinal pre-alpha cell
	clusters
Jeste & Lohr (1989)	Reduction of hippocampal volume and pyr-
	amidal cell numbers

and interpeduncular nucleus are damaged by a cut separating right from left hemispheres, and only very few right hemispheres are available.

To overcome these methodological problems, we started in 1984 at the Department of Psychiatry, University of Düsseldorf, to collect new brains of 40 clinically well-diagnosed schizophrenic patients and 60 control cases without neurological or psychiatric diseases. Meanwhile, volume measurements of the whole hippocampal formation by planimetry of 20-micrometer myelin- and Nissl-stained serial sections of 20 schizophrenics and 20 well-matched controls have been finished. The mean hippocampal volume on the right and the left side was highly significantly reduced by about 20%; the whole length of the hippocampus measured from the level of the splenium of the corpus callosum up to the anterior pole of the hippocampus was also significantly reduced by about 15%; whereas the mean cross-sectional areas were unchanged. We interpreted the reduced length of the hippocampus as a failure of development to its final anterior position.

An outstanding result of these more recent studies is that all qualitative and quantitative post-mortem investigations of the medial temporal lobe structures (i.e. hippocampal formation including the dentate gyrus, para-hippocampal gyrus which contains in part the entorhinal cortex, amygdala) and of the cingulate gyrus (which is functionally closely related to them) found structural abnormalities of one or several of these limbic brain parts in a substantial proportion of schizophrenics (see Table 8.1 and Table 8.2). Nearly all of these studies, however, have some of the above-mentioned methodological and statistical problems, which are inherent in post-mortem human brain morphometry, and suffer from small sample sizes, and some from poorly-matched controls. It is remarkable, however, that all studies that investigated limbic structures of schizophrenics came to the conclusion that there are structural abnormalities. As of now, there have been no post-mortem studies on limbic brain regions of schizophrenics that were unable to detect histopathological changes in these pivotal brain parts. I think it is justified to state that limbic system pathology has become one of the most frequently replicated findings in biological studies of schizophrenia. The fate of morphological schizophrenia research during the first half of this century has not seemed to repeat itself.

Until the first half of the century, the limbic system was widely regarded as being a part of the olfactory system. Hence, before then, neuropathologists had no special interest in these structures; they were therefore generally overlooked in the search for pathomorphological substrata of schizophrenia.

Can schizophrenic symptoms be related to the reported brain anomalies?

Our present knowledge of brain anatomy and physiology allows an attempt to explain why limbic dysfunctions are associated with schizophrenic symptoms.

Figure 8.1 shows a very simplified schematic diagram of the neuroanatomy of information processing. All visual, auditory and somatosensory inputs to the neocortex follow a cascade-like arrangement of information processing from the primary visual, auditory and somatic sensory cortical regions to unimodal association areas surrounding the primary sensory cortical areas. After a first analysis in the unimodal association cortex, sensory input is transferred to polymodal association areas, which integrate two or more sensory modalities, and from there to the supramodal association cortex where all sensory modalities are integrated at a high neuronal level. The paralimbic brain regions such as orbital cortex, cingulate gyrus, temporal pole and parahippocampal gyrus are to be regarded as highly-organized supramodal association and integration areas (Jones & Powell, 1970; Swanson, 1983; Mesulam, 1986; Schmajuk, 1987). It seems reasonable to

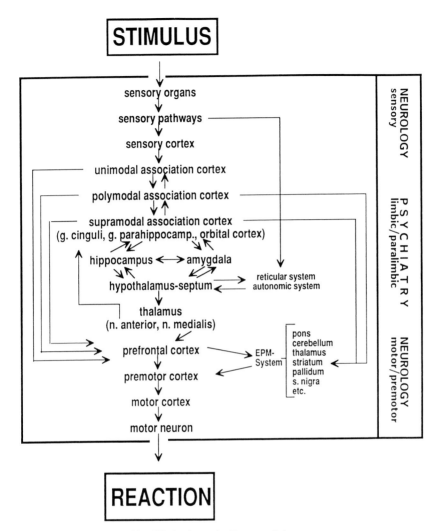

Figure 8.1. Simplified schematic diagram of the neuroanatomical pathways underlying cerebral information processing. The schema demonstrates that limbic and paralimbic structures are anatomically and functionally interposed between sensory and motor or autonomic brain regions. Limbic/paralimbic brain regions are also the only structures that link neocortical cognitive activities to phylogenetically old drives and emotions generated in the septum–hypothalamus complex. (For further explanations see text.)

assume that structural and functional deficits in these brain regions are associated with the failure of many schizophrenics in the higher integrative and associative brain functions, leading to distorted interpretations of the external reality (Torrey & Peterson, 1974; Bogerts et al., 1987; Bogerts, 1989).

Figure 8.1 further demonstrates that hippocampus and amygdala, which are the central limbic structures of the temporal lobe, are anatomically and functionally interposed between the supramodal sensory associations areas on the one side and the septum–hypothalamus complex on the other side. All sensory information finally converges in the hippocampus and amygdala, which are key structures in sensory information processing (Jones and Powell, 1970; Mesulam, 1986). Hippocampus and amygdala also play an important role in the so-called 'sensory gating', which is the filtering out of irrelevant sensory stimuli by the neuronal comparison of present with past experience.

Furthermore, amygdala and hippocampus control by several fiber bundles the phylogentically old basic drives and emotions that are generated in neuronal networks of the septum–hypothalamus complex. Thus, in addition to disturbed sensory information processing, limbic pathology could also explain the dyscontrol syndrome of basic emotions that is frequently seen in schizophrenics (Bogerts, 1985, 1988, 1989).

Since the amygdala, hippocampus and entorhinal cortex (and to some extent the orbital cortex, too) are structures that link the neocortical sensory association areas with the septum–hypothalamus complex, and since there are no direct connections between neocortex and hypothalamus (Swanson, 1983; Palkovits & Zaborsky, 1979), structural and functional disturbances of these pivotal structures lead to a dissociation between neocortical–cognitive activities and hypothalamic–emotional reactions to these activities. This dissociation – which induced Bleuler (1911) to coin the term 'schizophrenia' – may result in an inappropriate emotional categorization of sensory percep-tions, and hence to a disturbed experience of the external reality (Bogerts, 1988, 1989).

Motor reactions to environmental stimuli analyzed and processed by paralimbic and limbic structures can be modulated from there via hypo-thalamus, medial thalamus, prefrontal and premotor cortex; autonomic nervous system responses via hypothalamus and lower brainstem structures. Thus, the limbic and paralimbic telencephalic and diencephalic structures shown in the middle third of Figure 8.1 can be regarded as an interface between sensory cortical systems on the one hand and motor/autonomic systems on the other hand. Lesions of the motor and sensory brain parts, which are shown in the upper and lower third of Fig. 8.1, are regularly associated with well-defined neurological syndromes; whereas lesions of limbic and paralimbic structures and related diencephalic brain regions are known to cause syndromes that are frequently indistinguishable from the so-called endogenous psychoses (Davison & Bagley, 1969).

It is an important principle in neurology that the clinical picture of neurological syndromes depends on the site and not on the nature or etiology of the lesion. The pathomorphological findings in schizophrenia and organic schizophrenia-like psychoses (Davison & Bagley, 1969; Hillbom, 1951), and the pathophysiological considerations discussed above, support the notion that the same principle can be applied in psychiatry; this means that: (1) psychiatric diseases occur if higher brain systems structurally and functionally interposed between motor and sensory systems are affected; (2) the type of psychopathology depends on the site within the brain where the structural or functional disturbance occurs, but not on how the lesion was caused.

According to this point of view, to explain the pathophysiology of psychotic symptoms it is unimportant whether prenatal, perinatal or early postnatal developmental disturbances, viral infections, autoimmunological processes, degenerative changes or anything else causes the anatomical anomalies and the resulting psychotic symptoms. The fact is decisive that limbic or paralimbic structures, or functional systems closely related to them, are disturbed.

Morphological changes have not only been described in limbic regions; they have also been described in the central thalamic cell group and diencephalic periventricular gray matter (Lesch & Bogerts, 1984), globus pallidus (Stevens, 1982; Bogerts et al., 1985), corpus callosum (Nasrallah et al., 1983, Bigelow et al., 1983) prefrontal cortex (Benes, Davidson & Bird, 1986) and catecholaminergic brainstem systems (Bogerts et al., 1983a; Lohr & Jeste, 1988), indicating that the neuromorphological alterations are not only confined to limbic brain regions but are more widespread and inhomogeneous, and may vary from patient to patient. The periventricular gray matter plays an important role in the integration of central vegetative functions; shrinkage of this tissue layer might be related to the vegetative symptoms frequently observed in schizophrenics (Huber, 1981; Lesch & Bogerts, 1984); pathology of the pallidum, which is a part of the extrapyramidal system, could be related to motor or catatonic symptoms of schizophrenics (Stevens, 1982, 1986). If the reported anomalies in structures situated outside the limbic system can be confirmed by future investigations, the inhomogeneous and varying neuropathology could be regarded as the morphological basis of various clinical subgroups of the disease.

How can abnormal brain morphology be related to the typical course of the disease?

As early as 1970 Mednick proposed that hippocampal pathology caused by genetic factors and/or pre- and perinatal complications could create a predisposition to adult schizophrenia. Histological findings consistent with this view were first reported by McLardy (1974). Most subsequent post-mortem studies agree that the structural abnormalities in limbic brain regions, such as smaller volumes of amygdala, entorhinal cortex and hippocampus, and reduced nerve cell numbers and cellular disarray in the hippocampus, dentate gyrus, entorhinal and cingulate cortex, are not due to an ongoing and progressive degenerative brain disease. The findings are rather suggestive of a disturbance of normal brain development occurring very early in childhood, possibly in the prenatal or perinatal period.

Lack of gliosis and cytoarchitectonic disturbances in the medial temporal lobe and cingulate gyrus, shape abnormalities of the hippocampus, and the absence of a significant correlation between structural alterations and disease duration in CT scans of schizophrenics (Shelton & Weinberger, 1986; Bogerts et al., 1987) indicate that, in at least a significant percentage of patients, the extent of limbic pathology remains stable during the whole life. Therefore, it is very likely that hypoplasias or dysplasias, but not atrophic processes, are the underlying neuropathological changes that cause a lifelong reduced functional capacity of the affected limbic and paralimbic structures. Smaller volumes, therefore, can be regarded as vulnerability markers rather than as state variables by which the typical course of the disease could be explained.

A static structural defect alone cannot explain the following characteristic features of the disease course: the time of onset of the typical schizophrenic symptoms, which is usually not before puberty; the periodic course, with relapses and recoveries; the decline of positive symptoms during old age; and the exacerbation of symptoms under stress. Therefore, additional factors have to be postulated, which lead to a functional decompensation of hypoplastic limbic structures in the vulnerable life period between puberty and old age, and in stress situations.

There are several theories that offer an explanation for the long latency between the assumed early occurrence of neuropathological abnormalities of schizophrenics and the onset of the typical clinical symptoms.

Weinberger (1987) proposed that the late appearance of schizophrenic symptoms is linked to the normal maturation of brain areas affected by early developmental pathology, particularly the dorsolateral prefrontal cortex. He related the course of the illness and the importance of stress to normal maturational aspects of dopaminergic neural systems innervating the prefrontal cortex. A similar theory, based on reports of developmental disturbances of hippocampus and associated cortex, was put forward by Murray *et al.* (1990). They assumed that neural dysplasia results in premorbid cognitive symptoms and negative schizophrenic symptoms whereas brain maturation changes in adolescence, possibly myelination or synaptic pruning, render the patients susceptible to hallucinations and delusions.

An alternative theory emphasizing hormonal developments during puberty has been published by us (Bogerts, 1987, 1988, 1989). Within the brain, limbic structures during puberty become the main targets of age- and stress-related hormones such as gonadosteroids and corticosteroids. It is conceivable that vulnerable (i.e. hypoplastic) limbic structures decompensate under the influence of such hormones, leading to psychotic symptoms.

Final confirmation or refutation of all of these hypotheses by empirical data is still lacking. The search for biological factors responsible for the considerable delay between onset of neuropathology and onset of the disease will be an important task for future research.

References

Altshuler, L., Conrad, A., Kovelman, J. A. & Scheibel, A. (1987). Hippocampal Pyramidal Cell Orientation in Schizophrenia. *Archives of General Psychiatry*, **44**, 1094–8.

Altshuler, L., Casanova, M. E., Goldberg, T. & Kleinman, J. (1988). Shape and area measurements of hippocampus and parahippocampal gyrus in schizophrenics, suicide and normal control brains. *Neuroscience Abstracts*, Nov. 1988.

Averback, P. (1981). Lesions of the nucleus ansae peduncularis in neuropsychiatric disease. *Archives of Neurology*, **38**, 230–5.

Benes, F. M. (1987). An analysis of the arrangement of neurons in the cingulate cortex of schizophrenic patients. *Archives of General Psychiatry*, **44**, 608–16.

Benes, F. M., Davidson, B. & Bird, E. D. (1986). Quantitative cytoarchitectural studies of the cerebral cortex of schizophrenics. *Archives of General Psychiatry*, **43**, 31–5.

Bigelow, L. B., Nasrallah, H. A. & Rauscher, F. P. (1983). Corpus callosum thickness in chronic schizophrenia. *British Journal of Psychiatry*, **142**; 282–7.

Bleuler, E. (1911). Dementia praecox oder die Gruppe der Schizophrenien. In G. Aschaffenburg (ed.) *Handbuch der Psychiatrie*, Vol. 4, pp. 230–85. Leipzig: Deuticke.

Bogerts, B. (1984). Zur Neuropathologie der Schizophrenien. *Fortschritte der Neurologie Psychiatrie*, **52**, 428–37.

(1985). Schizophrenien als Erkrankungen des limbischen Systems. In G. Huber (Ed.), *Basisstadien endogener Psychosen und das Borderline-Problem.* (pp. 163–79). Stuttgart: Schatteuer.

(1987). Interaktion von alters- und stressabhängigen Faktoren mit limbischen

Strukturdefiziten bein Schizophrenen. In H. Beckmann, G. Laux (Eds.) Biologische Psychiatrie, Synopsis 1986/87. Springer: Berlin, pp. 3–7.

(1988). Limbische und paralimbische Strukturdefekte als Trait-Marker schizophrener Erkrankungen – eine Integration neuroanatomischer, neuroradiologischer und klinischer Daten. In G. Oepen (Ed.), *Psychiatrie des rechten und linken Gehirns*, Deutscher Aerzte Verlag.

(1989). Limbic and paralimbic pathology in schizophrenia: Interaction with age and stress related factors. In S. C. Schulz & C. A. Tamminga (Eds.), *Schizophrenia: scientific progress*, (pp. 216–26). Oxford: Oxford University Press.

Bogerts, B., Falkai, P. & Tutsch, J. (1986). Cell numbers in the pallidum and hippocampus of schizophrenics. In: C. Shagass *et al.* (Eds.) *Biological Psychiatry*. (pp. 1178–80). Amsterdam: Elsevier.

Bogerts, B., Häntsch, J. & Herzer, M. (1983a). A morphometric study of the dopamine containing cell groups in the mesencephalon of normals, Parkinson patients and schizophrenics. *Biological Psychiatry*, **18**, 951–60.

Bogerts, B., Lesch, A., Lange, H., Zech, M. & Tutsch, J. (1983b). Hypotrophy of the corpus callosum in schizophrenia. *Neuroscience Letters* (suppl 14) abstract S34.

Bogerts, B., Meertz, E. & Schonfeld-Bausch, R. (1985). Basal ganglia and limbic system pathology in schizophrenia. *Archives of General Psychiatry*, **42**, 784–91.

Bogerts, B., Wurthmann, C. & Piroth, H. D. (1987). Hirnsubstanzdefizit mit paralimbischem und limbischem Schwerpunkt im CT Schizophrener. *Nervenarzt*, **58**, 97–106.

Brown, R., Colter, N., Corsellis, J. A. N., Crow, T. J., Frith, C. D., Jagoe, R., Johnstone, E. C. & Marsh, L. (1986). Postmortem evidence of structural brain changes in schizophrenia. Differences in brain weight, temporal horn area and parahippocampal gyrus compared with affective disorder. *Archives of General Psychiatry*, **43**, 36–42.

Casanova, M., Stevens, J. R. & Bigelow, L. (1987). Gliosis in schizophrenia. *Biological Psychiatry*, **22**, 1172–5.

Colter, N., Battal, S., Crow, T. J., Johnstone, E. C., Brown, R. & Bruton, C. (1987). White matter reduction in the parahippocampal gyrus of patients with schizophrenia. *Archives of General Psychiatry*, **44**, 1023.

Crow, T. J. (1985). The two-syndrome concept. Origins and current status. *Schizophrenia Bulletin*, **11**, 471–86.

David, G. B. (1957). The pathological anatomy of the schizophrenias. In: D. Richter (Ed.), *Schizophrenia: somatic aspects*, (pp. 93–130). London: Pergamon Press.

Davison, K. & Bagley, C. R. (1969). Schizophrenia-like psychosis associated with organic disorders of the central nervous system. A review of the literature. In: R. N. Hertington (ed.), *Current Problems in Neuropsychiatry*. British Journal of Psychiatry Special Publication No. 4: pp. 113–87.

Dom, R., de Saedeler, J., Bogerts, B. & Hopf, A. (1981). Quantitative cytometric analysis of basal ganglia in catatonic schizophrenics. In Perris *et al.* (Eds.), *Biological Psychiatry*, (pp. 723–6). Amsterdam: Elsevier.

Falkai, P. & Bogerts, B. (1986). Cell loss in the hippocampus of schizophrenics. *European Archives of Psychiatry and Neurological Sciences*, **236**, 154–61.

Falkai, P., Bogerts, B. & Rozumek, M. (1988a). Cell loss and volume reduction in the entorhinal cortex of schizophrenics. *Biological Psychiatry*, **24**, 515–21.

Falkai, P., Bogerts, B., Roberts, G. W. & Crow, T. J. (1988b). Measurement of the alpha-cell-migration in the entorhinal region: a marker for developmental disturbances in schizophrenia? *Schizophrenia Research*, 1, 157–8.

Fisman, M. (1975). The brain stem in psychosis. *British Journal of Psychiatry*, **126**, 414–22.

Greenough, W. T. & Zuraske, J. M. (1979). Experience induced changes in brain fine structure: their behavioural implications. In M. E. Hahn, C. Jensen & B. C. Dudex (eds.) pp. 295–320. New York: Academic Press.

Huber, G. (1981). *Psychiatrie*, 3rd edition. Stuttgart: Schattauer.

Jacobi, W. & Winkler, H. (1927). Encephalographische Studien an chronisch Schizophrenen. *Archiv für Psychiatrie und Nerven-Krankheiten*, **81**, 229–332.

Jakob, H. (1979). *Die Picksche Krankheit. Eine neuropathologisch–anatomisch–klinische Studie.* Berlin, Heidelberg, New York: Springer.

Jakob, J. & Beckmann, H. (1986). Prenatal developmental disturbances in the limbic allocortex in schizophrenics. *Journal of Neural Transmission*, **65**, 303–26.

Jeste, D. V. & Lohr, J. B. (1989). Hippocampal pathologic findings in schizophrenia, *Archives of General Psychiatry*, **46**, 1019–24.

Jones, E. G. & Powell, T. P. S. (1970). An anatomical study of converging sensory pathways within the cerebral cortex of the monkey. *Brain*, **93**, 793–820.

Kirch, D. & Weinberger, D. R. (1986). Anatomical neuropathology in schizophrenia: post mortem findings. In: H. A. Nasrallah & D. R. Weinberger (Eds.), *The neurology of schizophrenia*, (pp. 325–48). New York: Elsevier.

Kovelman, J. A. & Scheibel, A. B. (1984). A neurohistological correlate of schizophrenia. *Biological Psychiatry*, **19**, 1601–21.

(1986). Biological substrates of schizophrenia. *Acta Neurologica Scandinavica*, **73**, 1–32.

Larroche, J. L. (1984). Malformations of the nervous system. In J. M. Adams *et al.* (Eds.), *Greenfield's Neuropathology*, (pp. 385–403). London: Edward Arnold.

Lesch, A. & Bogerts, B. (1984). The diencephalon in schizophrenia: Evidence for reduced thickness of the periventricular grey matter. *European Archives of Psychiatry and Neurological Sciences*, **234**, 212–19.

Lohr, J. B. & Jeste, D. V. (1988). Locus ceruleus morphometry in aging and schizophrenia. *Acta Psychiatrica Scandinavica*, **77**, 689–97.

McLardy, T. (1974). Hippocampal zinc and structural deficit in brains from chronic alcoholics and some schizophrenics. *Journal of Orthomolecular Psychiatry*, **4** (1), 32–6.

Mednick, S. A. (1970). Breakdown in individual at high risk for schizophrenia. *Mental Hygiene*, **54**, 50–67.

Mesulam, M. M. (1986). Patterns in behavioral neuroanatomy: association areas, the limbic system, and hemispheric specialization. In: M. M. Mesulam, *Principles of behavioral neurology*, (pp. 1–70). Philadelphia: Davis.

Murray, R. M., Lewis, S. W., Owen, M. J. & Foerster, A. (1990). The neurodevelopmental origins of dementia praecox. In P. McGuffin, & P. Bebbington (Eds.), *Schizophrenia; the major issues.* London: Heinemann.

Nasrallah, H. A., Bigelow, L. B., Rauscher, F. P. & Wyatt, R. J. (1979). Corpus callosum thickness in schizophrenia. *New Research Abstracts* 15, American Psychiatric Association 132nd Annual Convention.

Nasrallah, H. A., McCalley-Whitters, M., Rauscher, F. P. *et al.* (1983). A histological study of the corpus callosum in chronic schizophrenia. *Psychiatry Research*, **8**, 151–60.

Nieto, D. & Escobar, A. (1972). Major psychoses. In J. Minkler (Ed.), *Pathology of the nervous system.* (pp. 2654–65). New York: McGraw-Hill.

Oyanagi, K., Yoshida, Y. & Icuta, F. (1986). The chronology of lesion repair in the developing rat brain. *Virchows Archiv (Pathologische Anatomie)*, pp. 347–59.

Pakkenberg, B. (1987). Post-mortem study of chronic schizophrenic brains. *British Journal of Psychiatry*, **151**, 744–52.

Palkovits, M. & Zaborsky, L. (1979). Neural connections of the hypothalamus. In P. J. Morgane (Ed.), *Anatomy of the hypothalamus.* (pp. 379–509). New York: Decker.

Papez, J. W. (1937). A proposed mechanism of emotion. *Archives of Neurology and Psychiatry*, **38**, 725–43.

Peters, G. (1967). Neuropathologie und Psychiatrie. In H. W. Gruhle, R. Jung, W. Mayer-Gross & M. Müller (Eds.). *Psychiatrie der Gegenwart*, (pp. 286–98). Berlin: Springer.

Roberts, G. W., Colter, N., Lofthouse, R., Bogerts, B., Zech, M. & Crow, T. J. (1986). Gliosis in schizophrenia: A survey. *Biological Psychiatry*, **21**, 1043–50.

Roberts, G. W., Colter, N., Lofthouse, R., Johnstone, E. C. & Crow, T. J. (1987). Is there gliosis in schizophrenia? Investigations of the temporal lobe. *Biological Psychiatry*, **22**, 1409–68.

Roberts, G. W. & Crow, T. J. (1987). The neuropathology of schizophrenia – a progress report. *British Medical Bulletin*, **43**(3), 599–615.

Rosenthal, R. & Bigelow, L. B. (1972). Quantitative brain measurements in chronic schizophrenia. *British Journal of Psychiatry*, **121**, 259–64.

Scheibel, A. B. & Kovelman, J. A. (1981). Disorientation of the hippocampal pyramidal cells and its processes in the schizophrenic patient. *Biological Psychiatry*, **16**, 101–2.

Schmajuk, N. A. (1987). Animal models for schizophrenia: the hippocampally lesioned animal. *Schizophrenia Bulletin*, **13**(2), 317–27.

Shelton, R. C. & Weinberger, D. R. (1986). X-ray computerized tomography studies in schizophrenia: a review and synthesis. In H. A. Nasrallah & D. R. Weinberger, *The Neurology of schizophrenia*, (pp. 207–50). New York: Elsevier.

Stevens, C. D., Altshuler, L. L., Bogerts, B. & Falkai, P. (1988). Quantitative study of gliosis in schizophrenia and Huntington's chorea. *Biological Psychiatry*, **24**, 697–700.

Stevens, J. R. (1982). Neuropathology of schizophrenia. *Archives of General*

Psychiatry, **39**, 1131–9.

(1986). Clinicopathological correlations in schizophrenia. *Archives of General Psychiatry*, **43**, 715–16.

Stevens, J. R., Casanova, M. & Bigelow, L. (1988). Gliosis in schizophrenia. *Biological Psychiatry*, **24**, 721–34.

Swanson, L. W. (1983). The hippocampus and the concept of limbic system. In W. Seifert (Ed.), *Neurobiology of the hippocampus.* (pp. 3–19). London: Academic Press.

Torrey, E. F. & Peterson, M. R. (1974). Schizophrenia and the limbic system. *Lancet*, **2**, 942–6.

Vogt, O. (1925). Der Begriff der Pathoklise. *Journal für Psycholgie und Neurologie*, **31**, 245–55.

Vogt, C. & Vogt, O. (1948). Über anatomische Substrate. Bemerkungen zur pathoanatomischen Befunden bei Schizophrenie. *Arztliche Forschung*, **3**, 1–7.

Walsh, R. N. (1981). Effects of environmental complexity and deprivation on brain anatomy and histology: a review. *International Journal of Neuroscience*, **12**, 33–51.

Weinberger, D. R., Wagner, R. L. & Wyatt, R. J. (1983). Neuropathological studies of schizophrenia: a selective review. *Schizophrenia Bulletin*, **9**, 193–212.

Weinberger, D. R. (1987). Implications of normal brain development for the pathogenesis of schizophrenia. *Archives of General Psychiatry*, **44**, 660–9.

9

Genetic and perinatal sources of structural brain abnormalities in schizophrenia

TYRONE D. CANNON

University of Southern California

Introduction

Modern brain imaging studies have found robust evidence of structural brain abnormalities in schizophrenic patients. The most widely replicated anomalies are cortical abnormalities and enlargement of the third and lateral ventricles. A major issue in evaluating the possible etiological significance of structural brain deficits in schizophrenia is whether the abnormalities reflect developmental disturbances associated with genetic and perinatal factors (e.g. Cannon, Mednick & Parnas, 1989) or a deteriorating process associated with advancing age, increasing length of illness, or repeated treatments with invasive physical therapies (Jellinek, 1976; Marsden, 1976; Trimble & Kingsley, 1978; Woods & Wolf, 1983). Another important etiological issue is whether the brain abnormalities are related to behavioral and phenomenological aspects of the disorder.

This chapter reviews evidence bearing on the possible neurodevelopmental and pathophysiological significance of abnormal brain imaging findings in schizophrenia. Three basic issues are addressed: (1) do the abnormalities deteriorate in the course of illness?; (2) do the abnormalities reflect disturbances of brain development?; and (3) do the abnormalities underlie important clinical features of the illness?

Deterioration

It is well known that, in normals, ventricular size tends to increase with age (Barron *et al.*, 1976). There is no reason to believe that aging factors do not also influence ventricular size in schizophrenics. However, since most of the brain imaging studies used age-matched control samples, it is unlikely that aging processes alone can explain the finding of structural brain pathology in schizophrenia. A more critical question is whether aspects of the schizo-phrenic disease process are also capable of influencing ventricular size. The variable typically used to index such processes is duration of illness. Duration of illness tends to be correlated with exposure to invasive physical treatments and presumably with any progressive aspects of the disease process in schizophrenia. As a temporal measure, duration of illness also tends to be highly correlated with age. Five studies reported significant correlations between duration of illness and lateral-ventricular size in their schizophrenic samples. Interestingly, in four of these five studies there was also a significant correlation between lateral ventricular enlargement and age (Andreasen et al., 1982; Mathew et al., 1985; Naber et al., 1985; Shima et al., 1985). This result suggests that the association between ventricular enlargement and duration of illness may not be independent of age. Two studies which examined this implication statistically found that duration of illness made a negligible and nonsignificant contribution to ventricular size once age was controlled (Andreasen et al., 1982; Mathew et al., 1985).

To determine whether duration of illness makes a significant contribution to ventricular size in the total population of schizophrenics examined in brain imaging studies, the mean age, mean duration of illness, and mean ventricle–brain ratio of the schizophrenic sample from each study was tabulated; these values were then subjected to correlational analysis across studies. The mean ventricle–brain ratio of the schizophrenic samples was significantly correlated with their mean age ($r = 0.60$, $n = 66$ studies, $p < 0.0001$) (see Fig. 9.1) and mean length of illness ($r = 0.46$, $n = 47$, $p < 0.0001$). After controlling for the relationship between ventricle–brain ratio and age, the correlation between ventricle–brain ratio and duration of illness was reduced and became nonsignificant ($r = 0.09$, $n = 47$, ns). The mean age and ventricle–brain ratio of the control samples were also significantly correlated, to about the same degree as in the schizophrenic samples: $r = 0.55$, $n = 50$, $p < 0.0001$ (see Fig. 9.1). The distribution of ventricle–brain ratios for younger schizophrenics is similar to that of normals who are several decades older.

It is important to note that relationships between variables at the level of sample means do not necessarily reflect relationships between those variables at the level of individuals. Nevertheless, the findings reported above are consistent with the results of similar analyses conducted on individual data (Andreasen et al., 1982; Mathew et al., 1985), and the shapes of the ventricle–brain ratio distributions are remarkably similar to those obtained in individual studies (e.g. Barron, Jacobs & Kinkel, 1976; Pearlson et al., 1989).

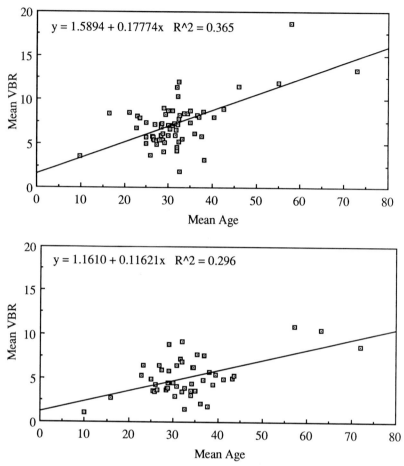

Figure 9.1. Mean ventricle–brain ratios (VBRs) of 66 schizophrenic samples (upper) and 50 control samples (lower) plotted against their mean ages.

Using this approach, increasing age accounts for about one-third of the variance in the mean ventricle–brain ratios of both schizophrenic and control samples, and duration of illness makes a negligible contribution to the schizophrenics' mean ventricle–brain ratios once aging variance is controlled.

Genetic and perinatal factors

While it is widely accepted that genetic and perinatal factors contribute substantially to the etiology of schizophrenia, the precise mechanisms are not well understood. Two competing hypotheses have been developed: (1) the *diathesis–stress* model, which suggests that genetic and environmental factors interact in the development of structural brain changes and later schizophrenia (e.g. Cannon, Mednick & Parnas, (1990a); and (2) the *familial–sporadic* model, which posits that where genetic predisposition is high, schizophrenia may develop without the presence of other factors, and where genetic predisposition is low, environmental factors are required to produce breakdown (e.g. Kendler & Hays, 1982; Lewis *et al.*, 1987).

Studies examining genetic and perinatal contributions to structural brain abnormalities in schizophrenia have used strategies that are differentially suited to test implications of the diathesis–stress and familial–sporadic models. The studies can be divided into four types: (1) comparisons among schizophrenics, their non-ill siblings or co-twins, and normal controls; (2) comparisons among high-risk offspring subdivided according to whether *one* or *both* of the parents are schizophrenic; (3) comparisons among unrelated schizophrenics subdivided on the basis of birth and family history; and (4) post-mortem neuropathology studies which examine the origins of brain abnormalities based on details of cell structure and orientation.

Family studies

The three studies that have compared the brain characteristics of schizophrenics with their normal siblings or co-twins and to normal controls have obtained remarkably consistent results, with each finding a significant familial contribution to ventricular size (DeLisi *et al.*, 1986; Reveley *et al.*, 1982; Weinberger *et al.*, 1981). Reveley *et al.* (1982) found that the heritability coefficients for ventricular area and ventricle–brain ratio were very high in both normal monozygotic twins (98%) and in monozygotic twins discordant for schizophrenia (87%). The schizophrenics had significantly greater ventricular areas and ventricle–brain ratios than their non-ill co-twins and the normal controls, and there was a nonsignificant trend for the co-twins to have larger ventricles than the controls. The higher ventricular values in the schizophrenics and their co-twins relative to controls could reflect the effects of either shared genes or shared environments, but the larger values in the schizophrenic twins relative to their co-twins must reflect differential environments, since their genetic compositions are identical. In the Weinberger *et al.* (1981) study, schizophrenics and their non-ill siblings evidenced significantly larger ventricles than normal controls, indicating a common genetic–familial component to increased ventricular size. In this study the schizophrenics also had significantly larger ventricles than their non-ill *siblings* (i.e. not twins), which could reflect a higher genetic loading, differential environmental conditions, or both. DeLisi *et al.* (1986) examined the contributions of birth and family variables to ventricular enlargement in 26 schizophrenics and 10 non-ill siblings from 12 different families and 20 normal controls. Birth complications were assessed using a standardized questionnaire filled out by the mother of each subject. Birth complications accounted for the largest amount of variance in ventricular size (34%), but both family membership and diagnostic status were significantly related to ventricular size even after controlling for the effects of birth complications, age, and head injuries. This finding suggests that there is a significant association between ventricular size and schizophrenia *within families* even after the contributions of several environmental causes are partialled out. Unfortunately, the overlap (i.e. interaction) in the contributions of family membership and obstetric complications was not assessed.

High-risk studies

Only one prospective high-risk study has examined structural abnormalities in relation to genetic and perinatal antecedent factors. All of the subjects in this study had schizophrenic mothers; thus, the major source of genetic variability was determined by the diagnostic status of their fathers. The fathers were interviewed blindly with respect to offspring diagnosis and brain morphology and were assigned lifetime DSM-III (i.e. according to the Diagnostic and Statistical Manual of Mental Disorders, Version III) diagnoses. It was found that genetic and perinatal factors were differentially related to the various brain regions examined: (1) cortical and cerebellar abnormalities formed a single factor which was predicted by the presence of schizophrenia-spectrum disorder in the subjects' fathers (R-square $= 0.17$) but was not related to prospectively-assessed pregnancy or delivery complications or to weight at birth; (2) third and lateral ventricular enlargement formed a separate factor that was predicted primarily by the *interaction* of genetic risk for schizophrenia and complications of delivery (R-square $= 0.49$) (Cannon *et al.*, 1989). This study provides the most direct support for a joint genetic–perinatal determination of ventricular enlargement in schizophrenia. It should be noted, however, that the study design did not permit examination of the effects of obstetric complications in the absence of some degree of genetic risk.

Unselected samples

Family history. Studies examining genetic and perinatal contributions to brain morphology using unselected samples of schizophrenics have obtained inconsistent results. Six studies which used family history as a factor were excluded from the review because they failed to specify the diagnostic criteria or procedures and/or the definition of a positive family history (Boronow *et al.*, 1985; Kemali *et al.*, 1985; Owens *et al.*, 1985; Romani *et al.*, 1986; Tanaka *et al.*, 1981; Williams *et al.*, 1985). Of the remaining 13 studies, three found larger ventricles in patients without a positive family history (Cazullo, Vita & Sacchetti, 1989; Reveley, Reveley & Murray, 1983; Turner, Toone & Brett-Jones, 1986), two found larger ventricles in patients with a positive history (Kaiya *et al.*, 1989; Nasrallah *et al.*, 1983a), and eight found no relationship (Campbell *et al.*, 1979; Farmer *et al.*, 1987; Nasrallah *et al.*, see Chapter 11; Nimgaonkar, Wessely & Murray, 1988; Owen, Lewis & Murray, 1990; Pandurangi *et al.*, 1986; Pearlson *et al.*, 1985; Pearlson *et al.*, 1989). In the Nasrallah *et al.* study (see Chapter 11), a positive family history for schizophrenia was significantly associated with reduced cranial, cerebral, and frontal area as assessed on magnetic resonance imaging (MRI) scan. This finding is consistent with their earlier hypothesis that reduced cranial, cerebral, and frontal size may reflect 'early developmental abnormality' associated with genetic and/or perinatal influences (Andreasen *et al.*, 1986). Supportive evidence was found by two studies (DeLisi *et al.*, 1986; Kaiya *et al.*, 1989), but not by two others (DeLisi *et al.*, 1985; Oxenstierna *et al.*, 1984). In an MRI study, DeLisi, Dauphinais & Gershon (1988) found high sib-pair correlations for volume of the total limbic complex, right anterior gyrus and left posterior hippocampus, which may suggest a heritable component to the decreased size of these structures in schizophrenics as compared with controls. However, there were no differences in subcortical pathology as a function of delivery complications in this small group of patients.

Obstetric history. Five studies that used obstetric history as a factor were excluded from the review because they failed to specify how obstetric complications were assessed and/or how positive obstetric complication histories were defined (Boronow *et al.*, 1985; Cazullo *et al.*, 1989; Kemali *et al.*, 1985; Owens *et al.*, 1985; Williams *et al.*, 1985). Of the remaining eleven studies, five found that history of obstetric complications was positively related to increased ventricular size (Lewis & Murray, 1987; Owen, Lewis & Murray, 1988; Pearlson *et al.*, 1985; Pearlson *et al.*, 1989; Turner *et al.*, 1986), one found a negative correlation between obstetric complications and ventricle–brain ratio (Kaiya *et al.*, 1989), and five did not find significant correlations between ventricular enlargement and birth history in the schizophrenic samples (Nasrallah *et al.*, see Chapter 11; Nimgaonkar *et al.*, 1988; Oxenstierna *et al.*, 1984; Reveley *et al.*, 1983; Reveley, Reveley & Murray, 1984). In three studies there was a dissociation between family history and obstetric history, supporting the familial–sporadic model (Cazullo *et al.*, 1989; Nasrallah *et al.*, see Chapter 11; Reveley *et al.*, 1983).

Methodological flaws. The inconsistent results of studies using unselected samples are not surprising in view of their questionable methodological foundations. The major limitation of the family history design is that dividing patients into family history positive and negative groups fails to account for false negatives due to small family size, evasion of the diagnostic process, or failure of expression of genetic vulnerability (DeLisi *et al.*, 1986). Many of these studies are also vulnerable to an excessive rate of false positives (DeLisi *et al.*, 1985; Nimgaonkar *et al.*, 1988; Owen *et al.*, 1990; Oxenstierna *et al.*, 1984; Pearlson *et al.*, 1985; Reveley *et al.*, 1983, 1984), since positive family history was defined as the presence of *any* major psychiatric disorder in the family, which is a dubious basis from which to infer genetic risk for *schizophrenia*. The findings with respect to obstetric history are limited primarily by the use of retrospective, nonuniform, and nonstandardized assessment procedures. In some of the studies (i.e. Reveley *et al.*, 1983; 1984; Turner *et al.*, 1986) birth complications were assessed only by interview of the patient. The major limitation with respect to the finding of dissociation between family and obstetric history is that the sources of the information for the two variables were often the *same*, which opens the possibility for selective or biased recall or reporting based on 'pet' hypotheses of the cause of illness or explanations that exonerate the reporter from blame. This process could systematically and artefactually dissociate positive family and obstetric histories in view of the fact that the subject's mother was most frequently the source of the family and birth information.

Continuity of ventricle–brain ratio distribution

Weinberger (1987, 1989) has argued that since the majority of CT and MRI studies have not found evidence of a bimodal distribution of ventricular values in schizophrenics but, rather, a positively skewed, unimodal distribution, ventricular enlargement in schizophrenia may reflect a more homogeneous underlying pathological process than is usually assumed. That is, since there is a large degree of normal variability in brain morphology and in the morphology that would be expected for schizophrenics, the upwardly skewed distribution in schizophrenia may indicate that most if not all schizophrenics suffer from varying degrees of the same underlying process. Weinberger (1989) has suggested that normal siblings or co-twins are the most appropriate controls for schizophrenics in brain imaging studies because they provide a more accurate estimate of the values that would be expected for the schizophrenics if they did not suffer from the disorder. In support of this hypothesis, the National Institute of Mental Health (NIMH) group reported results from a study of monozygotic twins discordant for schizophrenia. In all or nearly all of the cases, the schizophrenic twin was found to evidence larger third and lateral ventricles (on MRI scan) and lower frontal-lobe activation during the Wisconsin Card Sorting Test (as assessed by positron emission tomography (PET) scan) than their non-ill co-twin (Suddath *et al.*, 1990). It is important to note, however, that studies using interfamilial designs do not support the hypothesis of a homogeneous underlying pathological process. Since in all of these studies schizophrenics had larger ventricular values than their sibs, who in turn tended to have larger values than nonrelated controls, genetic factors alone may be one source of increased ventricular size in schizophrenia, while genetic and environmental factors combined may explain another share of the increases. This point does not, however, dispute the overall upward shift in the distribution of ventricular values in schizophrenics or the importance of controlling for biological heterogeneity by using relatives of schizophrenics as one form of control.

Post-mortem studies

Post-mortem neuropathology studies have also examined the pathogenesis of brain deficits in schizophrenia. While none of these studies attempted to correlate brain abnormalities with family or birth variables, several reported evidence of cellular disturbances consistent with genetic or teratogenic disruptions of fetal neural development. This evidence includes disorientation of hippocampal pyramidal cells (Kovelman & Scheibel, 1984), disturbed migration or lamination of cells in the basal ganglia (Bogerts, Meerts & Schonfeldt-Bausch, 1985) and entorhinal cortex (Jakob & Beckmann, 1986), disturbed cell arrangements in the cingulate cortex (Benes & Bird, 1987), and ventricular widening in the absence of significant gliosis (Crow *et al.*, 1989). In two of these reports the evidence was said to be consistent with developmental disturbances in the second trimester gestation, when these brain regions undergo maximal growth (Jakob & Beckmann, 1986; Kovelman & Scheibel, 1984). Since viral infection in the second trimester has been linked to an increased risk for later schizophrenia (Barr, Mednick & Munk-Jorgensen, in press; Mednick *et al.*, 1988), viral agents and other teratogens represent one possible source for the fetal neural developmental anomalies. Another possible source is genetic factors. Rakic and Sidman (1973) and Nowakowski (see Chapter 4) have each postulated and confirmed that genetic factors can produce errors of cell migration in inbred strains of mice.

Clinical correlates

If the brain abnormalities observed in schizophrenics play an etiological role in the disorder, then they should be related to important aspects of the clinical presentation of these patients and should help to explain the heterogeneity of symptoms.

Premorbid functioning

One important implication of an early (i.e. gestational or perinatal) origin of the brain abnormalities in schizophrenia is that they may be associated with behavioral, cognitive, and other disturbances *early* in life. All three of the reports using prospective assessment of premorbid functioning have come from the Copenhagen schizophrenia high-risk project (Mednick & Schulsinger, 1965). In one report, lateral ventricular enlargement in adulthood was significantly associated with a stable pattern of impaired scholastic and occupational functioning from age 15 to age 25 (Erel *et al.*, 1990). In two other reports, third ventricular enlargement in adulthood was significantly related to reduced electrodermal responsiveness (Cannon *et al.*, 1988) and heart-rate activity (Cannon *et al.*, 1990b) in adolescence.

One retrospective study was located which defined premorbid adjustment on the basis of scholastic history. In this study, ventricular enlargement in adulthood was related to academic difficulties during elementary and secondary education (Pearlson *et al.*, 1985). The other retrospective studies are difficult to interpret because none is based on uniform, objective records and because retrospective assessments based on recall of the patient, parents, or other informants are not very reliable. In view of these considerations, it is not surprising that retrospective studies have obtained conflicting results. Three studies using either the Phillips or Cannon–Spoor premorbid adjustment scales found significant relationships between ventricular enlargement and impaired premorbid functioning (DeLisi *et al.*, 1983; Jeste *et al.*, 1982; Weinberger *et al.*, 1980); six other studies failed to replicate these findings (Andreasen *et al.*, 1982; Boronow *et al.*, 1985; DeLisi *et al.*, 1986; Kemali *et al.*, 1985; Pandurangi *et al.*, 1986; van Kammen *et al.*, 1983). In addition, two studies which used ratings of 'schizoid traits' found significant relationships between premorbid social impairment and ventricular enlargement (Pearlson *et al.*, 1985; Williams *et al.*, 1985).

Neuropsychological deficits

Neuropsychological tests. Over 40 studies were located that examined the relationship between brain morphology and cognitive functioning in schizophrenic samples. Half of these studies employed full test-battery assessments such as the Luria-Nebraska Neuropsychological Battery (LNNB) and the Halstead-Reitan Neuropsychological Battery (HRNB). Five out of seven studies that examined performance on the LNNB in patients with and without structural brain deficits (primarily ventricular enlargement) found that the CT-positive patients were significantly more impaired (Cazullo *et al.*, 1989; Golden *et al.*, 1980a; 1980c; 1982; Kemali *et al.*, 1985). About 80% of the patients could be classified correctly into CT-positive and CT-negative groups on the basis of their LNNB profiles alone (Golden *et al.*, 1980a; 1980b; 1982). Most of the misclassified cases were in the CT-normal group. With respect to localization, one study (Kemali *et al.*, 1985) found a significant correlation between ventricular enlargement and the left (but not right) hemisphere scale of the LNNB, suggesting a left-hemisphere focus of pathology. In two studies by Golden *et al.* (1980c; 1982), ventricle–brain ratio was either equally correlated or equally uncorrelated with the left and right hemisphere scales. However, patients with enlarged ventricles were consistently found to show deficits on scales requiring *language* skills. In another study by Golden and colleagues (1981), significant left-hemisphere density deficits were noted in a sample of 23 chronic schizophrenic patients selected because of impairment on the LNNB. Unfortunately, no effort was made in this study to relate individual LNNB subtests to either global or regional density values. Two studies failed to find a relationship between LNNB performance and CT scan deficits (Carr & Wedding, 1984; Pfefferbaum *et al.*, 1988). In the Carr and Wedding (1984) study, all of the schizophrenics were severely cognitively impaired. Curiously, although the schizophrenics had larger ventricles than the controls, the ventricle–brain ratios of both groups were much smaller than those found by other investigators and the ranges were restricted, suggesting measurement error and/or a homogeneous patient sample with uniformly enlarged ventricles.

Twelve of the 16 studies that examined performance on the HRNB and/or Wechsler Adult Intelligence Scale (WAIS) in schizophrenics with and without abnormal CT scans found significantly more impairment in patients with some form of structural abnormality (primarily third and lateral ventricular enlargement, but also reduced cerebral and cranial size) (Adams, Jacism & Brown, 1980; Andreason *et al.*, 1986; Bilder *et al.*, 1988; Boucher *et al.*, 1986; Cazullo *et al.*, 1989; Donnelley *et al.*, 1980; Jeste *et al.*, 1982; Katsanis & Iacono, 1989; Lawson, Waldman & Weinberger, 1988; Nyman *et al.*, 1986; Pandurangi *et al.*, 1986; Reider *et al.*, 1979). Six of the 12 studies reporting positive findings examined relationships between structural deficits and specific subtests of the HRNB. In general, the findings suggested deficits in language functions, cognitive flexibility, attention, memory, and sensory–perceptual integration (Andreason *et al.*, 1986; Donnelly *et al.*, 1980; Katsanis & Iacono, 1989; Lawson *et al.*, 1988; Nyman *et al.*, 1986). In one study, third but not lateral ventricular enlargement was related to a pattern of deficits suggestive of left hemisphere pathology (Nyman *et al.*, 1986). In nine of the 12 studies reporting positive findings, one or more of the HRNB summary scores correctly classified between 70% and 90% of the patients with and without abnormal CT signs, with most of the misclassified cases coming from the CT-normal group. There was an overall trend for the Halstead Impairment Index to be superior in this discrimination to other summary indices (i.e. Percentage of Ratings in the Impaired Range and Average Impairment Rating). Performance on the WAIS was less consistently related to structural abnormalities than was performance on the HRNB (Bankier, 1985; Bilder *et al.*, 1988; Boronow *et al.*, 1985; Boucher *et al.*, 1986; Cazullo *et al.*, 1989; DeMeyer *et al.*, 1984; Donnelley *et al.*, 1980; Kemali *et al.*, 1985; Lawson *et al.*, 1988, Nyman *et al.*, 1986; Pandurangi *et al.*, 1986; Seidman *et al.*, 1987; Vita *et al.*, 1988; Weinberger *et al.*, 1979). Four studies failed to find a relationship between structural abnormalities and cognitive impairment using the HRNB and/or WAIS (Bankier, 1985; Carr & Wedding, 1984; DeMeyer *et al.*, 1984; Weinberger *et al.*, 1979). In one case the IQ tests were performed before the study began, for clinical reasons, suggesting probable selection bias (Weinberger *et al.*, 1979); in another case the patient sample included patients with several psychiatric disorders, not just schizophrenia (DeMeyer *et al.*, 1984); and in another case ventricular size was assessed by ultrasound (Bankier, 1985), which is of unknown reliability and may not be directly comparable with CT and MRI assessments.

Overall, the evidence strongly supports an association between structural brain abnormalities and neuropsychological deficits in schizophrenia. However, since structural abnormalities may contribute to a more chronic, treatment-resistant condition, it is important to assess the role of secondary factors which may mediate this association. Potential secondary factors include age, gender, educational history, neuroleptic and anticholinergic medications, electro-convulsive therapy, hospitalization, psychiatric symptoms such as apathy and anergia, and other factors which are known to affect cognitive performance (Frith, 1984; Jellinek, 1976; Marsden, 1976; Perlick *et al.*, 1986). Only seven studies examined brain deficits in relation to specific cognitive functions, were apparently free of sampling and/or selection biases, and ruled out the effects of mediating variables including age, education, duration of illness, neuroleptic medications, and hospitalization. All seven of these *relatively* methodologically sound studies found evidence of a relationship between structural brain abnormalities and neuropsychological impairment (Andreasen *et al.*, 1986; Golden *et al.*, 1980b,c; Golden *et al.*, 1982; Katsanis & Iacono, 1989; Kemali *et al.*, 1985; Donnelley *et al.*, 1980; Lawson *et al.*, 1988; Nyman *et al.*, 1986). Limitations of these studies include the use of mostly male patient groups and the failure to control for movement disorders, anticholinergic medications, or clinical symptomatology.

In two controlled studies, schizophrenics with and without enlarged ventricles evidenced a similar pattern of cognitive deficits, but the patients with enlarged ventricles were relatively more impaired (Kemali *et al.*, 1985; Lawson *et al.*, 1988). This pattern is consistent with the continuum of pathology concept advocated by Weinberger (1989). According to this view, all schizophrenics have varying degrees of structural abnormalities when intra- and interfamilial variability in brain morphology is accounted for; thus, if structural abnormalities are the basis of cognitive dysfunction in schizophrenia, all schizophrenics would be expected to evidence varying degrees of the *same* types of neuropsychological impairments.

Bilder *et al.* (1988) examined the relationship between lateral ventricular enlargement and performance on tests assessing 'hold' and 'don't hold' cognitive abilities. They suggested that ventricular enlargement may be more associated with a pattern indicative of cognitive deterioration than of impaired premorbid ability. However, studies examining neuropsychological characteristics of schizophrenic patients longitudinally have failed to find evidence of a deteriorating process (Seidman, 1983; Waddington & Youssef, 1989), suggesting that their underlying causes are stable and not progressive. These findings are consistent with studies reviewed previously which point to an early (i.e. gestational or perinatal) pathogenesis of the brain abnormalities in schizophrenia and which suggest a lack of progression beyond that associated with normal aging processes.

Mental status assessments. Studies that examined the relationship between structural brain abnormalities and cognitive impairment using mental status assessments obtained mixed results. Five studies found a positive association between ventricular enlargement and impaired mental status (Johnstone *et al.*, 1976; 1978; Andreasen *et al.*, 1982; Goldberg *et al.*, 1988; Nasrallah *et al.*, 1983b), while six studies failed to replicate these findings (Famiyuwa *et al.*, 1979; Kolakowska *et al.*, 1985; Kling *et al.*, 1983; Nasrallah *et al.*, 1983a; Owens *et al.*, 1985; Pearlson *et al.*, 1989). In part, the lack of convergence reflects several methodological inadequacies of these studies, including nonrandom selection (Johnstone *et al.*, 1976, 1978), scoring of mental status from nonuniform case records (Nasrallah *et al.*, 1983a,b), and the use of unspecified, qualitative scoring criteria for the CT scans (Famiyuwa *et al.*,

185

1979). The discrepant findings may also reflect the fact that mental status assessments are less sensitive to subtle and/or specific cognitive deficits than are neuropsychological test batteries.

Hypofrontal blood flow. Berman *et al.* (1987) found a correlation between lateral ventricular enlargement and reduced blood flow to the prefrontal cortex during the Wisconsin Card Sorting Task, a neuropsychological test designed specifically to activate frontal regions. Interestingly, another study failed to find a relationship between prefrontal *structural* pathology and impaired performance on the Wisconsin card sort (Andreasen *et al.*, 1986). Together, these findings suggest that deficits in 'frontal' cognitive activities (e.g. planning, organization, learning from experience, solving problems, introspection) may be based on *functional* but not structural abnormalities of the prefrontal cortex, which in turn may be secondary to subcortical pathology and/or disturbances in subcortical–cortical projection systems (Berman *et al.*, 1987).

EEG disturbances. Studies examining structural abnormalities in relation to electroencephalographic deficits are of variable quality. Both studies that used a standard stimulus presentation paradigm and also provided details of the scoring procedures found significant associations between structural abnormalities and changes in evoked potential responses at specific latencies (McCarley *et al.*, 1989; Morihisa & McAnulty, 1985). Of the remaining studies, two reported relationship between lateral ventricular enlargement and EEG slowing (Karson, Coppola & Daniel, 1988; Pandurangi *et al.*, 1986), while two others failed to find relationships between ventricular enlargement and unspecified 'EEG abnormalities' (Boronow *et al.*, 1985; Oxenstierna *et al.*, 1984).

Eye movement dysfunctions. Two studies examined lateral ventricular enlargement in relation to eye-movement dysfunctions. Bartfai *et al.* (1985) found a nonsignificant trend toward larger anterior horn widths in patients with deviant eye-tracking, but there was no relationship between smooth pursuit eye movement (SPEM) abnormalities and third ventricle width. Cazullo *et al.* (1989) found *more* SPEM abnormalities in patients *without* evidence of ventricular enlargement on CT scan. Unfortunately, neither study attempted to assess abnormalities in the cerebellar vermis region. It has been suggested that dysgenesis of the vermis may be a genetically-mediated deficit underlying some of the SPEM dysfunctions observed in schizophrenics and their relatives (Cannon *et al.*, 1989).

Clinical symptomatology

The considerable variability in clinical symptomatology among schizophrenic patients suggests that schizophrenia may represent a heterogeneous
group of disorders. In view of this heterogeneity, it has been suggested that
biological findings such as ventricular enlargement may help to define
specific etiological and phenomenological subtypes (e.g. Crow, 1980). While
many approaches to subtyping have been suggested, the subtyping system
that has received much attention in the last decade of schizophrenia research
is based on the distinction between negative and positive symptoms.
Negative symptoms include flat affect, anergia, anhedonia-asociality, and
attentional impairment. Positive symptoms include hallucinations, delusions, and thought disorder.

Negative and positive symptoms. Studies examining the association between
ventricular enlargement and negative symptoms have obtained mixed
results. In nine studies, schizophrenics with enlarged ventricles were found
to evidence significantly more negative symptoms than schizophrenics
without enlarged ventricles (Besson *et al.*, 1987; Cazullo *et al.*, 1989; Kaiya *et
al.*, 1989; Kemali *et al.*, 1985; Moscarelli *et al.*, 1989; Owens *et al.*, 1985;
Pearlson *et al.*, 1985; Seidman *et al.*, 1987; and Williams *et al.*, 1985).
However, 15 other studies failed to confirm these results (Andreasen *et al.*,
1982; Bishop *et al.*, 1983; Boronow *et al.*, 1985; DeLisi *et al.*, 1986; Johnstone
et al., 1976; Losonczy *et al.*, 1986; Luchins, Lewine & Meltzer, 1984;
Mathew *et al.*, 1985; Naber *et al.*, 1985; Nasrallah *et al.*, 1983a; Ota *et al.*,
1987; Pandurangi *et al.*, 1986; Pearlson *et al.*, 1989; Pfefferbaum *et al.*, 1988;
and Shelton *et al.*, 1988).

There are two primary explanations for the discrepant findings of these
studies. First, some of the studies that failed to find relationships between
ventricular enlargement and negative symptoms used items or factor scores
from the Brief Psychiatric Rating Scale (Bishop *et al.*, 1983; Boronow *et al.*,
1985; Naber *et al.*, 1985; and Shelton *et al.*, 1988). The Brief Psychiatric
Rating Scale is a general, all-purpose instrument for the assessment of
psychopathology; discriminant and conconcurrent validity studies with
respect to the negative symptom construct have not been conducted. If only
those studies using scales designed and validated specifically for the
assessment of negative symptoms were considered (i.e. Scale for the
Assessment of Negative Symptoms [Andreasen & Olsen, 1982] and
Krawiecka scales [Krawiecka, Goldberg & Vaughn, 1977]), a larger percentage of studies (i.e. 50%) found relationships between ventricular enlargement and negative symptoms.

Second, while some studies using validated scales failed to find significantly more negative symptoms in schizophrenics with enlarged ventricles, several did find significantly fewer positive symptoms in these patients (Andreasen *et al.*, 1982; Luchins *et al.*, 1984; Ota *et al.*, 1987; Pearlson *et al.*, 1989). These results suggest that a more useful approach is to consider structural abnormalities in relation to predominantly negative and positive forms of schizophrenia. One study that examined an index of relative symptomatology found that patients with enlarged ventricles had more negative symptoms relative to positive symptoms than patients with narrow ventricles (Andreasen *et al.*, 1982). While none of the remaining studies examined the issue of relative symptomatology directly, many found negative correlations between ventricular enlargement and positive symptoms. Eleven out of 15 studies (73%) using validated symptom scales found that patients with enlarged ventricles evidenced more negative symptoms or fewer positive symptoms, or both, compared with patients with narrow ventricles. It is also important to note that no study found more positive symptoms in patients with enlarged ventricles.

Diagnostic subtypes. There is no consistent pattern of correlation between brain abnormalities and traditional diagnostic subtypes. Six studies reported that patients with subtype diagnoses in the residual, hebephrenic, undifferentiated, or 'Kraepelinian' categories had larger ventricles than patients with subtype diagnosis in the paranoid or acute categories (Frangos & Athanassenas, 1982; Kling *et al.*, 1983; Losonczy *et al.*, 1986; Luchins & Meltzer, 1986; Nasrallah *et al.*, 1982a; Tachiki *et al.*, 1984); five studies found no relationship between ventricular enlargement and subtype diagnoses (Bishop *et al.*, 1983; Cazullo *et al.*, 1989; Golden *et al.*, 1980c; Owens *et al.*, 1985; Weinberger *et al.*, 1979); and two other studies found larger ventricles in patients with paranoid or 'positive' subtype diagnoses (Farmer *et al.*, 1987; Nasrallah *et al.*, 1982b).

Conclusion

The major competing hypothesis to the view that structural brain abnormalities are involved in the etiology of schizophrenia is that many of the deficits could be consequences of aging and illness processes (e.g. Jellinek, 1976; Marsden, 1976; Trimble & Kingsley, 1978; Woods & Wolf, 1983). Correlational analysis of sample characteristics across studies found that age accounted for about one-third of the variance in lateral ventricular size in *both* schizophrenics and controls, and that duration of illness made a negligible contribution to the schizophrenics' ventricle–brain ratios once aging variance was controlled statistically. Together, these findings suggest strongly that ventricular enlargement in schizophrenia is not progressive beyond that associated with *normal* aging processes.

Since secondary factors probably do not explain a major share of the structural abnormalities found in schizophrenics, it seems likely that at least some of the abnormalities are associated with the etiology of schizophrenia. Studies using high-risk and interfamilial designs found consistent evidence of both genetic–familial and environmental–perinatal contributions to brain abnormalities in schizophrenics (Cannon *et al.*, 1989; DeLisi *et al.*, 1986; Reveley *et al.*, 1982; Weinberger *et al.*, 1981). Examination of the relationship between different types of abnormalities in terms of their etiological antecedents suggested that while generalized developmental abnormalities in cortical and cerebellar regions were associated with genetic risk for schizophrenia, third and lateral ventricular enlargement were predicted primarily by the interaction of genetic risk for schizophrenia and complications of delivery (Cannon *et al.*, 1989). Neuropathology studies also observed two primary types of structural abnormalities: (1) gestational disturbances in various regions of the cortex and limbic system (Benes & Bird, 1987; Bogerts *et al.*, 1985; Jakob & Beckmann, 1986; Kovelman & Scheibel, 1984); and (2) periventricular tissue damage, particularly in the region of the third ventricle (e.g. Lesch & Bogerts, 1984; Nieto & Escobar, 1972; Stevens, 1982). The nature and location of the gestational abnormalities suggests some type of disturbance in the second trimester of gestation (Jakob & Beckmann, 1986; Kovelman & Scheibel, 1984). Both genetic (see Chapter 4) and teratogenic (e.g. viral: Kendell & Kemp, 1989; Mednick *et al.*, 1988) contributions to the gestational disturbances are possible.

Together, these findings support a gene–environment interaction hypothesis: (1) the genetic predisposition to schizophrenia may be expressed as a disruption of fetal brain development, perhaps centered in the second trimester of gestation; (2) in individuals with the genetically-based fetal neural developmental deficits, anoxia and/or hemorrhage secondary to complications at birth may produce increased periventricular tissue damage, which in turn may increase the likelihood of overt schizophrenia (Cannon, Mednick & Parnas, 1989; 1990; Mednick *et al.*, 1988).

An important test of the role of brain abnormalities in the etiology of schizophrenia is whether or not they underlie clinical features of the illness. Prospective evidence supports an association between third and lateral ventricular enlargement and deficits in premorbid autonomic and scholastic functioning (Cannon *et al.*, 1988, 1990b; Erel *et al.*, 1990). The strongest evidence for a pathogenic role of the brain abnormalities in schizophrenia is the relationship between structural deficits and neuropsychological functioning. In studies using full test-battery assessments, structural abnormalities (primarily third and lateral ventricular enlargement, but also reduced cerebral and cranial size) were consistently related to cognitive impairments, particularly with respect to language and sensory–perceptual functions. Studies relating structural abnormalities such as ventricular enlargement to physiological deficits such as reduced prefrontal blood flow and autonomic responsiveness appear to have the greatest potential for localizing the deficits relevant to the pathophysiology of schizophrenia. Preliminary evidence suggests that these physiological and information-processing deficits may be mediated by subcortical changes in areas around the ventricular system, such as the thalamus, hypothalamus, and other mesolimbic structures (Berman et al., 1987; Cannon et al., 1988, 1990b).

The case for a specific clinical sybtype based on underlying structural pathology is mixed. Neuropsychological impairments are not unique to schizophrenics with abnormal brain scans; however, the degree of cognitive impairment does appear to covary with the degree of structural damage. Similarly, the evidence does not support a clear distinction between negative and positive forms of schizophrenia, but it is consistent with the view that structural abnormalities are more common (or apparent) in patients with predominantly negative symptoms and a relative lack of positive symptoms.

Acknowledgements

Preparation of this chapter was supported by a National Research Service Award from the National Institute of Mental Health.

References

Adams, K. M., Jacism, J. & Brown, G. G. (1980). Neuropsychological and CT deficits in schizophrenics. Paper presented at the 133rd Annual American Psychiatric Association meeting, San Francisco.

Andreasen, N. C., Nasrallah, H. A., Dunn, V., Olson, S. C., Grove, W. M., Ehrhardt, J. C., Coffman, J. A. & Crossett, J. H. W. (1986). Structural abnormalities in the frontal system in schizophrenia. *Archives of General Psychiatry*, **43**, 136–44.

Andreasen, N. C. & Olsen, S. A. (1982). Negative v positive schizophrenia: Definition and validation. *Archives of General Psychiatry*, **39**, 789–94.

Andreasen, N. C., Olsen, S. A., Dennert, J. W. & Smith, M. R. (1982). Ventricular enlargement in schizophrenia: Relationship to positive and negative symptoms. *American Journal of Psychiatry*, **139**, 297–302.

Bankier, R. G. (1985). Third ventricle size and dementia in schizophrenia. *British Journal of Psychiatry*, **147**, 241–5.

Barr, C. E., Mednick, S. A. & Munk-Jorgensen, P. (1990). Exposure to influenza epidemics during gestation and adult schizophrenia: A 40 year study. *Archives of General Psychiatry*, **47**, 869–74.

Barron, S. A., Jacobs, L. & Kinkel, W. R. (1976). Changes in size of normal lateral ventricles during aging determined by computerized tomography. *Neurology*, **26**, 1011–13.

Bartfai, A., Levander, S. E., Nyback, H., Berggren, B.-M. & Schalling, D. (1985). Smooth pursuit eye-tracking, neuropsychological tests and computed tomography of the brain in schizophrenic patients. *Psychiatry Research*, **15**, 49–62.

Benes, F. M. & Bird, E. D. (1987). An analysis of the arrangement of neurons in the cingulate cortex of schizophrenic patients. *Archives of General Psychiatry*, **44**, 608–16.

Berman, K. F., Weinberger, D. R., Shelton, R. C. & Zec, R. F. (1987). A relationship between anatomical and physiological brain pathology in schizophrenia: Lateral cerebral ventricle size predicts cortical blood flow. *American Journal of Psychiatry*, **144**, 1277–82.

Besson, J. A. O., Corrigan, F. M., Cherryman, G. R. & Smith, F. W. (1987). Nuclear magnetic resonance brain imaging in chronic schizophrenia. *British Journal of Psychiatry*, **150**, 161–3.

Bilder, R. M., Degreef, G., Pandurangi, A. K., Rieder, R. O., Sackeim, H. A. & Mukherjee, S. (1988). Neuropsychological deterioration and CT scan findings in chronic schizophrenia. *Schizophrenia Research*, **1**, 37–45.

Bishop, R. J., Golden, C. J., MacInnes, W. D., Chu, C.-C., Ruedrich, S. L. & Wilson, J. (1983). The BPRS in assessing symptom correlates of cerebral ventricular enlargement in acute and chronic schizophrenia. *Psychiatry Research*, **9**, 225–31.

Bogerts, B., Meertz, E. & Schonfeldt-Bausch, R. (1985). Basal ganglia and limbic system pathology in schizophrenia: A morphometric study of brain volume and shrinkage. *Archives of General Psychiatry*, **42**, 784–91.

Boronow, J., Pickar, D., Ninan, P. T., Roy, A., Hommer, D., Linnoila, M. & Paul, S. M. (1985). Atrophy limited to the third ventricle in chronic schizophrenia. *Archives of General Psychiatry*, **42**, 266–71.

Boucher, M. J., Dewan, M. J., Donnelly, M. P., Pandurangi, A. K., Bartell, K., Diamond, T. & Major, L. F. (1986). Relative utility of three indices of neuropsychological impairment in a young, chronic schizophrenic population. *Journal of Nervous and Mental Disease*, **174**, 44–6.

Campbell, R., Hays, P., Russel, D. B. & Zacks, D. J. (1979). CT scan variants and genetic heterogeneity in schizophrenia. *American Journal of Psychiatry*, **136**, 722–3.

Cannon, T. D., Fuhrmann, M., Mednick, S. A., Machon, R. A., Parnas, J. & Schulsinger, F. (1988). Third ventricle enlargement and reduced electrodermal responsiveness. *Psychophysiology*, **25**, 153–6.

Cannon, T. D., Mednick, S. A. & Parnas, J. (1989). Genetic and perinatal determinants of structural brain deficits in schizophrenia. *Archives of General Psychiatry*, **46**, 883–9.

(1990a). Antecedents of predominantly negative and predominantly positive symptom schizophrenia in a high-risk population. *Archives of General Psychiatry*, **47**, 622–32.

Cannon, T. D., Raine, A., Herman, T. M., Mednick, S. A., Parnas, J., Schulsinger,

F. & Moore, M. (1990b). Third ventricle enlargement and reduced heart rate levels in a high-risk sample. *Psychophysiology*, in press.

Carr, E. G. & Wedding, D. (1984). Neuropsychological assessment of cerebral ventricular size in chronic schizophrenics. *International Journal of Clinical Neurology and Psychology*, **6**, 106–11.

Cazullo, C. L., Vita, A. & Sacchetti, E. (1989). Cerebral ventricular enlargement in schizophrenia: Prevalence and correlates. In S. C. Schulz & C. A. Tamminga (Eds.), *Schizophrenia: Scientific Progress* (pp. 195–206). New York: Oxford University Press.

Crow, T. J. (1980). Molecular pathology of schizophrenia: More than one disease process? *British Medical Journal*, **12**, 66–8.

Crow, T. J., Ball, J., Bloom, S. R., Brown, R., Bruton, C. J., Colter, N., Frith, C. D., Johnstone, E. C., Owens, D. G. C. & Roberts, G. W. (1989). Schizophrenia as an anomaly of development of cerebral asymmetry. *Archives of General Psychiatry*, **46**, 1145–50.

DeLisi, L. E., Buchsbaum, M. S., Halcomb, H. H., Dowling-Zimmerman, S., Pickard, D., Boronow, J., Morihisa, J. M., van Kammen, D. P., Carpenter, W., Kessler, R. & Cohen, R. M. (1985). Clinical correlates of decreased anteroposterior metabolic gradients. *American Journal of Psychiatry*, **142**, 78–81.

DeLisi, L. E., Goldin, L. R., Hamovit, J. R., Maxwell, E., Kurtz, D. & Gershon, E. S. (1986). A family study of the association of increased ventricular size with schizophrenia. *Archives of General Psychiatry*, **43**, 148–53.

DeLisi, L. E., Schwartz, C. C., Targum, S. D., Byrnes, S. M., Cannon-Spoor, E., Weinberger, D R. & Wyatt, R. J. (1983). Ventricular brain enlargement and outcome of acute schizophreniform disorder. *Psychiatry Research*, **9**, 169–71.

DeLisi, L. E., Dauphinais, I. D. & Gershon, E. S. (1988). Perinatal complications and reduced size of brain limbic structures in familial schizophrenia. *Schizophrenia Bulletin*, **14**, 185–91.

DeMeyer, M. K., Gilmor, R., DeMeyer, W. E., *et al.* (1984). Third ventricle size and ventricular–brain ratio in treatment-resistent psychiatric patients. *Journal of Operational Psychiatry*, **15**, 2–8.

Donnelley, E. F., Weinberger, D. R., Waldman, I. N., & Wyatt, R. J. (1980). Cognitive impairment associated with morphological brain abnormalities on computed tomography in chronic schizophrenic patients. *Journal of Nervous and Mental Disease*, **168**, 305–8.

Erel, O., Cannon, T. D., Hollister, M., Mednick, S. A. & Parnas, J. (1990). Ventricular enlargement and premorbid deficits in school–occupational attainment in a high-risk sample. *Schizophrenia Research*, in press.

Famiyuwa, O., Eccleston, D., Donaldson, A. & Garside, R. (1979). Tardive dyskinesia and dementia. *British Journal of Psychiatry*, **135**, 500–4.

Farmer, A., Jackson, R., McGuffin, P. & Storey, P. (1987). Cerebral ventricular enlargement in chronic schizophrenia: Consistencies and contradictions. *British Journal of Psychiatry*, **150**, 324–30.

Frangos, E. & Athanassenas, G. (1982). Differences in lateral brain ventricular size among various types of chronic schizophrenics. *Acta Psychiatrica Scandinavica*, **66**, 459–63.

Frith, C. D. (1984). Schizophrenia, memory, and anticholinergic drugs. *Journal of Abnormal Psychology*, **93**, 339–41.

Goldberg, T. E., Kleinman, J. E., Daniel, D. G., Myslobodsky, M. S., Ragland, J. D. & Weinberger, D. R. (1988). Dementia praecox revisited. Age disorientation, mental status, and ventricular enlargement. *British Journal of Psychiatry*, **153**, 187–90.

Golden, C. J., Graber, B., Coffman, J., Berg, R., Bloch, S. & Brogan, D. (1980a). Brain density deficits in chronic schizophrenia. *Psychiatry Research*, **3**, 179–84.

Golden, C. J., Graber, B., Coffman, J., Berg, R. A., Newlin, D. B. & Bloch, S. (1981). Structural brain deficits in schizophrenia: Identification by computed tomographic scan density measurements. *Archives of General Psychiatry*, **38**, 1014–17.

Golden, C. J., Graber, B., Moses, J. A. & Zatz, L. M. (1980b). Differentiation of chronic schizophrenics with and without ventricular enlargement by the Luria-Nebraska neuropsychological battery. *International Journal of Neuroscience*, **11**, 131–8.

Golden, C. J., MacInnes, W. D., Ariel, R. N., Reudrich, S. L., Chu, C. C., Coffman, J. A., Graber, B. & Bloch, S. (1982). Cross-validation of the ability of the Luria-Nebraska Neuropsychological Battery to differentiate chronic schizophrenics with and without structural abnormalities. *Journal of Consulting and Clinical Psychology*, **50**, 87–95.

Golden, C. J., Moses, J. A., Zelazowski, R., Graber, B., Zatz, L. M., Horvath, T. B. & Berger, P. A. (1980c). Cerebral ventricular size and neuropsychological impairment in young chronic schizophrenics. *Archives of General Psychiatry*, **37**, 619–23.

Jakob, H. & Beckmann, H. (1986). Prenatal-developmental disturbances in the limbic allocortex in schizophrenia. *Biological Psychiatry*, 1181–3.

Jellinek, E. H. (1976). Cerebral atrophy and cognitive impairment in chronic schizophrenia. *Lancet*, 1202–3.

Jeste, D. V., Kleinman, J. E., Potkin, S. G., Luchins, D. J. & Weinberger, D. R. (1982). *Ex uno multi*: Subtyping the schizophrenic syndrome. *Biological Psychiatry*, **17**, 199–222.

Johnstone, E. C., Crow, T. J., Frith, C. D., Husband, J. & Kreel, L. (1976). Cerebral ventricular size and cognitive impairment in chronic schizophrenia. *Lancet*, **1**, 924–6.

Johnstone, E. C., Crow, T. J., Frith, C. D., Stevens, M., Kreel, L. & Husband, J. (1978). The dementia of dementia praecox. *Acta Psychiatrica Scandinavica*, **57**, 305–24.

Kaiya, H., Uematsu, M., Ofuji, M., Nishida, A., Morikiyo, M. & Adachi, S. (1989). Computerised tomography in schizophrenia. Familial versus non-familial forms of illness. *British Journal of Psychiatry*, **155**, 444–50.

Karson, C. N., Coppola, R. & Daniel, D. G. (1988). Alpha frequency in schizophrenia: An association with enlarged cerebral ventricles. *American Journal of Psychiatry*, **145**, 861–4.

Katsanis, J. & Iacono, W. G. (1989). Association of left-handedness with ventricle size and neuropsychological performance in schizophrenia. *American Journal of Psychiatry*, **146**, 1056–8.

Kemali, D., Maj, M., Galderisi, S., Ariano, M. G., Cesarelli, M., Milici, N., Salvati, A., Valente, A. & Volpe, M. (1985). Clinical and neuropsychological correlates of cerebral ventricular enlargement in schizophrenia. *Journal of Psychiatric Research*, **19**, 587–96.

Kendell, R. E. & Kemp, I. W. (1989). Maternal influenza in the etiology of schizophrenia. *Archives of General Psychiatry*, **46**, 878–82.

Kendler, K. S. & Hays, P. (1982). Familial and sporadic schizophrenia: A symptomatic, prognostic and EEG comparison. *American Journal of Psychiatry*, **139**, 1557–62.

Kling, A. S., Kurtz, N., Tachiki, K. & Orzeck, A. (1983). CT scans in sub-groups of chronic schizophrenics. *Journal of Psychiatric Research*, **17**, 375–84.

Kling, A. S., Metter, E. J., Riege, W. H. & Kuhl, D. E. (1986). Comparison of PET measurement of local brain glucose metabolism and CAT measurement of brain atrophy in chronic schizophrenia and depression. *American Journal of Psychiatry*, **143**, 175–80.

Kolakowska, T., Williams, A. O., Ardern, M., Reveley, M. A., Jambor, K., Gelder, M. G. & Mandelbrote, B. M. (1985). Schizophrenia with good and poor outcome. I: Early clinical features, response to neuroleptics and signs of organic dysfunction. *British Journal of Psychiatry*, **146**, 229–38.

Kovelman, J. A. & Scheibel, A. B. (1984). A neurohistological correlate of schizophrenia. *Biological Psychiatry*, **19**, 1601–21.

Krawiecka, M., Goldberg, D. & Vaughn, M. (1977). A standardized psychiatric assessment scale for rating chronic psychotic patients. *Acta Psychiatrica Scandinavica*, **55**, 299–308.

Lawson, W. B., Waldman, I. N. & Weinberger, D. R. (1988). Schizophrenic dementia: Clinical and computed axial tomography correlates. *Journal of Nervous and Mental Disease*, **176**, 207–12.

Lesch, A. & Bogerts, B. (1984). The diencephalon in schizophrenia: Evidence for reduced thickness in the periventricular grey matter. *European Archives of Psychiatry and Neurological Sciences*, **234**, 212–19.

Lewis, S. W. & Murray, R. M. (1987). Obstetric complications, neurodevelopmental deviance, and risk of schizophrenia. *Journal of Psychiatric Research*, **21**, 413–21.

Lewis, S. W., Reveley, A. M., Reveley, M. A., Chitkara, B. & Murray, R. M. (1987). The familial–sporadic distinction as a strategy in schizophrenia research. *British Journal of Psychiatry*, **151**, 306–13.

Losonczy, M. F., Song, I. S., Mohs, R. C., Small, N. A., Davidson, M., Johns, C. A. & Davis, K. L. (1986). Correlates of lateral ventricular size in chronic schizophrenia, I: Behavioral and treatment response measures. *American Journal of Psychiatry*, **143**, 976–81.

Luchins, D. J. & Meltzer, H. Y. (1986). A comparison of CT findings in acute and chronic ward schizophrenics. *Psychiatry Research*, **17**, 7–14.

Luchins, D. J., Lewine, R. R. J. & Meltzer, H. Y. (1984). Lateral ventricular size, psychopathology, and medication response in the psychoses. *Biological Psychiatry*, **19**, 29–44.

Marsden, C. D. (1976). Cerebral atrophy and cognitive impairment in chronic schizophrenia. *Lancet*, **1**, 1079.

STRUCTURAL BRAIN ABNORMALITIES IN SCHIZOPHRENIA

Mathew, R. J., Partain, C. L., Rakash, R., Kulkarni, M. V., Logan, T. P. & Wilson, W. H. (1985). A study of the septum pellucidum and corpus callosum in schizophrenia with MR imaging. *Acta Psychiatrica Scandinavica*, **72**, 414–21.

McCarley, R. W., Faux, S. F., Shenton, M., LeMay, M., Cane, M., Ballinger, R. & Duffy, F. H. (1989). CT abnormalities in schizophrenia. A preliminary study of their correlations with P300/P200 electrophysiological features and positive/negative symptoms. *Archives of General Psychiatry*, **46**, 698–708.

Mednick, S. A. & Schulsinger, F. (1965). A longitudinal study of children with a high risk for schizophrenia: A preliminary report. In S. Vandenberg (Ed.), *Methods and goals in human behavior genetics* (pp. 255–96). New York: Academic Press.

Mednick, S. A., Machon, R. A., Huttunen, M. O. & Bonett, D. (1988). Adult schizophrenia following prenatal exposure to an influenza epidemic. *Archives of General Psychiatry*, **45**, 189–92.

Morihisa, J. M. & McAnulty, G. B. (1985). Structure and function: Brain electrical activity mapping and computed tomography in schizophrenia. *Biological Psychiatry*, **20**, 3–19.

Moscarelli, M., Cesana, B. M., Ciussani, S., Novti, N. C. & Cazullo, C. L. (1989). Ventricle–brain ratio and alogia in 19 young patients with chronic negative and positive schizophrenia. *American Journal of Psychiatry*, **146**, 257–8.

Naber, D., Albus, M., Burke, H., Muller-Spahn, F., Munch, U., Reinertshofer, T., Wissman, J. & Akenheil, M. (1985). Neuroleptic withdrawal in chronic schizophrenia, CT and endocrine variables relating to psychopathology. *Psychiatry Research*, **16**, 207–19.

Nasrallah, H. A., Jacoby, C. G., McCalley-Whitters, M. & Kuperman, S. (1982a). Cerebral ventricular enlargement in subtypes of chronic schizophrenia. *Archives of General Psychiatry*, **39**, 774–7.

Nasrallah, H. A., Rizzo, M., Damasio, H., McCalley-Whitters, M., Kuperman, S. & Jacoby, C. G. (1982b). Neurological differences between paranoid and non-paranoid schizophrenia: II. Computerized tomographic findings. *Journal of Clinical Psychiatry*, **43**, 307–9.

Nasrallah, H. A., Kuperman, S., Hamra, B. J. & McCalley-Whitters, M. (1983a). Clinical differences between schizophrenic patients with and without large cerebral ventricles. *Journal of Clinical Psychiatry*, **44**, 407–9.

Nasrallah, H. A., Kuperman, S., Jacoby, C. G., McCalley-Whitters, M. & Hamra, B. (1983b). Clinical correlates to sulcal widening in chronic schizophrenia. *Psychiatry Research*, **10**, 237–42.

Nieto, D. & Escobar, A. (1972). Major psychoses. In J. Minkerl (Ed.), *Pathology of the nervous system* (pp. 2654–65). New York: McGraw-Hill.

Nimgaonkar, V. L., Wessely, S. & Murray, R. M. (1988). Prevalence of familiality, obstetric complications, and structural brain damage in schizophrenic patients. *British Journal of Psychiatry*, **153**, 191–7.

Nyman, H., Nyback, H., Wiessel, G.-A., Oxenstierna, G. & Schalling, D. (1986). Neuropsychological test performance, brain morphological measures and CSF monoamine metabolites in schizophrenic patients. *Acta Psychiatrica Scandinavica*, **74**, 292–301.

Ota, T., Maeshiro, H., Ishido, H., Shimizu, Y., Uchida, R., Toyoshima, R., Ohshima, H., Takazawa, A., Motomura, H. & Noguchi, T. (1987). Treatment resistant chronic psychopathology and CT scans in schizophrenia. *Acta Psychiatrica Scandinavica*, **75**, 415–27.

Owen, M. J., Lewis, S. W. & Murray, R. M. (1988). Obstetric complications and schizophrenia: A computed tomographic study. *Psychological Medicine*, **18**, 331–9.

—— (1990). Family history and cerebral ventricular enlargement in schizophrenia: A case control study. *British Journal of Psychiatry*, in press.

Owens, D. G., Johnstone, E. C., Crow, T. J., Frith, C. D., Jagoe, J. R. & Kreel, L. (1985). Lateral ventricular size in schizophrenia: Relationship to the disease process and its clinical manifestations. *Psychological Medicine*, **15**, 27–41.

Oxenstierna, G., Bergstrand, G., Bjerkenstedt, L., Sedvall, G. & Wik, G. (1984). Evidence of disturbed CSF circulation and brain atrophy in cases of schizophrenic psychosis. *British Journal of Psychiatry*, **144**, 654–61.

Pandurangi, A. K., Dewan, M. J., Boucher, M., Levy, B., Ramachandran, T., Bartell, K., Bick, P. A., Phelps, B. H. & Major, L. (1986). A comprehensive study of chronic schizophrenic patients: II. Biological, neuropsychological, and clinical correlates of CT abnormality. *Acta Psychiatrica Scandinavica*, **73**, 161–71.

Pearlson, G. D., Garbacz, D. J., Moberg, P. J., Ahn, H. S. & DePaulo, J. R. (1985). Symptomatic, familial, perinatal, and social correlates of computerised axial tomography (CAT) changes in schizophrenics and bipolars. *Journal of Nervous and Mental Disease*, **173**, 42–50.

Pearlson, G. D., Kim, W. S., Kubos, K. L., Moberg, P. J., Jayaram, G., Bascom, M. J., Chase, G. A., Goldfinger, A. D. & Tune, L. E. (1989). Ventricle–brain ratio, computed tomographic density, and brain area in 50 schizophrenics. *Archives of General Psychiatry*, **46**, 690–7.

Perlick, D., Stastny, P., Katz, I., Mayer, M. & Mattis, S. (1986). Memory deficits and anticholinergic levels in chronic schizophrenia. *American Journal of Psychiatry*, **143**, 230–2.

Pfefferbaum, A., Zipursky, R. B., Lim, K. O., Zatz, L. M., Stahl, S. M. & Jernigan, T. L. (1988). Computed tomographic evidence for generalized sulcal and ventricular enlargement in schizophrenia. *Archives of General Psychiatry*, **45**, 633–40.

Rakic, P. & Sidman, R. L. (1973). Sequence of developmental abnormalities leading to granule cell deficit cerebellar cortex of weaver mutant mice. *Journal of Comparative Neurology*, **152**, 102–32.

Reider, R. O., Donnelley, E. F., Herdt, J. R. & Waldman, I. N. (1979). Sulcal prominence in young schizophrenic patients: CT scan findings associated with impairment on neuropsychological tests. *Psychiatry Research*, **1**, 1–8.

Reveley, A. M., Reveley, M. A., Clifford, C. A. & Murray, R. M. (1982). Cerebral ventricular size in twins discordant for schizophrenia. *Lancet*, **1**, 540–1.

Reveley, A. M., Reveley, M. A. & Murray, R. M. (1983). Enlargement of cerebral ventricles in schizophrenia is confined to those without known genetic predisposition. *Lancet*, **2**, 525.

—— (1984). Cerebral ventricular enlargement in nongenetic schizophrenia: A

controlled twin study. *British Journal of Psychiatry*, **144**, 89–93.
Romani, A., Zerbi, F., Mariotti, G., Callieco, R. & Cosi, V. (1986). Computed tomography and pattern reversal visual evoked potentials in chronic schizophrenic patients. *Acta Psychiatrica Scandinavica*, **73**, 566–73.
Seidman, L. J. (1983). Schizophrenia and brain dysfunction: An integration of recent neurodiagnostic findings. *Psychological Bulletin*, **94**, 195–238.
Seidman, L. J., Sokolove, R. L., McElroy, C., Knapp, P. H. & Sabin, T. (1987). Lateral ventricular size and social network differentiation in young, non-chronic schizophrenic patients. *American Journal of Psychiatry*, **144**, 512–14.
Shelton, R. C., Karson, C. N., Doran, A. R., Pickar, D., Bigelow, L. B. & Weinberger, D. R. (1988). Cerebral structural pathology in schizophrenia: Evidence for a selective prefrontal cortical defect. *American Journal of Psychiatry*, **145**, 154–63.
Shima, S., Kanba, S., Masuda, Y., Tsukomo, T., Kitamura, T. & Asai, M. (1985). Normal ventricles in chronic schizophrenics. *Acta Psychiatrica Scandinavica*, **71**, 25–29.
Stevens, J. R. (1982). Neuropathology of schizophrenia. *Archives of General Psychiatry*, **39**, 1131–9.
Suddath, R. L., Christison, D. A., Torrey, E. F., Casanova, M. F. & Weinberger, D. R. (1990). Anatomical abnormalities in the brains of monozygotic twins discordant for schizophrenia. *New England Journal of Medicine*, **322**, 791–4.
Tachiki, K. H., Kurtz, N., Kling, A. S. & Hullett, F. J. (1984). Blood monoamine oxidases and CT scans in subgroups of chronic schizophrenics. *Journal of Psychiatric Research*, **18**, 233–43.
Tanaka, Y., Hazama, H., Kawahara, R. & Kobayashi, K. (1981). Computerized tomography of the brain in schizophrenic patients. *Acta Psychiatrica Scandinavica*, **63**, 191–7.
Trimble, M. & Kingsley, D. (1978). Cerebral ventricular size in chronic schizophrenia. *Lancet*, 278–9.
Turner, S. W., Toone, B. K. & Brett-Jones, J. R. (1986). Computerized tomographic scan changes in early schizophrenia – preliminary findings. *Psychological Medicine*, **16**, 219–25.
van Kammen, D. P., Mann, L. S., Sternberg, D. E., Scheinin, M., Ninan, P. T., Marder, S. R., van Kammen, W., Rieder, R. O. & Linnoila, M. (1983). Dopamine-betahydroxylase activity and homvanillic acid in spinal fluid of schizophrenics with brain atrophy. *Science*, **220**, 974–7.
Vita, A., Sacchetti, E., Calzeroni, A. & Cazullo, C. L. (1988). Cortical atrophy in schizophrenia: Prevalence and associated features. *Schizophrenia Research*, **1**, 329–37.
Waddington, J. L. & Youssef, H. A. (1989). Cognitive function in schizophrenia followed prospectively over 5 years: Do neuropsychological deficits reflect active or static disease? *Paper presented at the Second International Congress on Schizophrenia Research*, San Diego, California, April 1–5, 1989.
Weinberger, D. R. (1987). Implication of normal brain development for the pathogenesis of schizophrenia. *Archives of General Psychiatry*, **44**, 660–9.
(1989). Clinical implications of temporal–prefrontal pathological findings in schizophrenia. *Paper presented at the Second International Congress on Schizophrenia Research*, San Diego, California, April 1–5, 1989.

Weinberger, D. R., Cannon-Spoor, E., Potkin, S. G. & Wyatt, R. J. (1980). Poor premorbid adjustment and CT scan abnormalities in chronic schizophrenia. *American Journal of Psychiatry*, **137**, 1410–13.

Weinberger, D. R., DeLisi, L. E., Neophytides, A. N. & Wyatt, R. J. (1981). Familial aspects of CT scan abnormalities in chronic schizophrenic patients. *Psychiatry Research*, **4**, 65–71.

Weinberger, D. R., Torrey, E. F., Neophytides, A. N. & Wyatt, R. J. (1979). Lateral cerebral ventricular enlargement in schizophrenia. *Archives of General Psychiatry*, **36**, 735–9.

Williams, A. O., Reveley, M. A., Kolakowska, T., Ardern, M. & Mandelbrote, B. M. (1985). Schizophrenia with good and poor outcome: II: Cerebral ventricular size and its clinical significance. *British Journal of Psychiatry*, **146**, 239–46.

Woods, B. T. & Wolf, J. (1983). A reconsideration of the relation of ventricular enlargement to duration of illness in schizophrenia. *American Journal of Psychiatry*, **140**, 1564–70.

10

Neurodevelopmental implications of findings from brain imaging studies of schizophrenia

NANCY A. BRESLIN AND DANIEL R. WEINBERGER

National Institute of Mental Health

Introduction

The application of so-called brain imaging techniques to the study of schizophrenia during the past thirteen years has had a dramatic impact on our understanding of this disorder. As compared with post-mortem studies, *in-vivo* neuroimaging presents a unique opportunity to study the brains of patients early in the course of illness, to study patients repeatedly, to collect more appropriate control data, and to avoid the numerous methodological pitfalls of post-mortem work. This body of research has resulted in the general acceptance of the existence of subtle cerebral morphological and physiological correlates of schizophrenia.

This chapter will discuss selected neuroimaging findings in the context of a neurodevelopmental approach to schizophrenia. From the earliest structural imaging studies of this illness, data emerged suggesting that the pathology involved is not adult in onset and is not degenerative. Most of the information collected to date is consistent with the notion that the structural abnormalities associated with schizophrenia are present at the onset of symptoms, probably were present early in life, and do not progress during the adult phase of illness. These data suggest a dissociation between the course of the development of the neuropathological correlates and the clinical course of the disorder. If this is so, it means that something else must interact with this pathology in order to account for the symptomatic course. It also means that the pathology can exist for relatively prolonged periods without producing an 'illness' and that the 'illness' appears and varies clinically without any change in the neuropathological substrate.

Table 10.1. *Elements of a neurodevelopmental model*

1. The pathology occurs and arrests early in nervous system development
2. The clinical manifestations of the pathology vary depending on ontogenic events that occur during normal brain development and on environmental factors

There are two essential components to the neurodevelopmental perspective as we see it: (1) the pathology itself occurs and arrests early in nervous system development; (2) the clinical ramifications of the pathological condition vary depending on independent ontogenic events that occur during normal brain development, and on environmental factors (Weinberger, 1987).

While this neurodevelopmental model of schizophrenia grew out of, rather than predated, recent neuroimaging research, one could have used it to make a number of predictions of what the various neuroimaging tools would show. First, the model would predict that, to the extent that gross neuropathology is present, it should be observed at the onset of the illness and should be found in some people who are at risk for the illness but who are as yet asymptomatic. Second, such changes should not vary with the length of illness. Third, the changes probably should correlate with some abnormal characteristics of premorbid behavior. Fourth, longitudinal studies should not find progression of neuropathology within individual patients. The results of studies of the influence of family history of illness or personal history of brain trauma would not necessarily be predicted by the model, as it does not attempt to explain the etiology for the pathology present, and various insults (trauma, genetic abnormality, infection) could account for the findings. Such studies could, however, lead to etiologic explanations. Each of these points will be considered in this chapter.

Review of brain imaging studies

General anatomical findings

Pneumoencephalography was the first *in-vivo* brain imaging technique available to neuroscientists. Developed in 1919, it was used in 1927 to study schizophrenic patients. While the technique was often painful and prone to technical errors (such as excessive injection of air artificially dilating the ventricular system), most of the results anticipated the findings that would be

Table 10.2. *Neuroimaging correlates of a neurodevelopmental model*

1. Pathology should be present at the onset of the illness and should be found in some people at risk for the illness but who are as yet asymptomatic
2. Evidence of pathology should not vary with the length of the illness
3. The pathological changes should probably correlate with some abnormal characteristics of premorbid behavior
4. Longitudinal studies should not find progression of neuropathology within individual patients

made later with non-invasive computerized tomography (CT) scanning. Haug (1962), Storey (1966) and Weinberger, Wagner & Wyatt (1983) review the work of pneumoencephalography in schizophrenia.

The first use of CT in schizophrenic patients was reported by Johnstone *et al.* in 1976, and soon replicated in a larger study of young patients by our own group (Weinberger *et al.*, 1979). In both studies, ventricular size was measured and found to be significantly larger in patients with schizophrenia as compared with normal volunteers. A number of reviews have recently been published that outline the findings of the first decade of CT work in schizophrenia (Shelton & Weinberger, 1986; Jaskiw, Andreasen & Weinberger, 1987; Andreasen, 1988). Shelton and Weinberger (1986) reviewed over 80 studies and noted that three-quarters of those that measured the lateral ventricles and over 80% of those that measured the third ventricle reported enlargement in schizophrenia. They attribute negative findings to three major factors: method of measurement, choice of control group, and patient selection. Linear measurements, the use of medical or neurological controls (Andreasen *et al.*, 1982), and the study of less-impaired patients, were all found to result in more frequently negative findings. Several papers suggest that volumetric measurement, rather than mechanical or digital planimetry, is even more sensitive to group differences (Reveley, 1985; Raz *et al.*, 1987).

In several studies, investigators have compared the CT scans of patients with schizophrenia with those of their healthy siblings. Weinberger *et al.* (1981), measuring ventricular sizes in the members of seven healthy sibships and ten containing at least one person with schizophrenia, found that while the ventricles of discordant siblings were all within the normal range, they were significantly larger than control values. Moreover, in each family the ill member had the largest ventricles. Reveley *et al.* (1982) scanned normal monozygotic and dizygotic twins and monozygotic pairs discordant for schizophrenia. They reported a high degree of heritability for ventricular size in all three groups, and in the discordant pairs the ill twins tended to have the larger ventricles. In a study by DeLisi *et al.* (1986), scans were done on ill and well members of twelve sibships. The patients with schizophrenia had larger ventricles than their siblings or controls, and a significant family component was again reported. These results suggest that subtle anatomical pathology may be a more consistent characteristic of patients with schizophrenia than has been inferred from population studies.

CT scans can yield additional structural information to that gained by ventricular measures. Sulcal widening, vermian changes, changes in tissue density, and abnormal cerebral asymmetries have also been studied, and are reviewed elsewhere (Shelton & Weinberger, 1986).

Using Magnetic Resonance Imaging (MRI), where ventricular size can be more accurately determined, results similar to the CT findings have emerged. Kelsoe *et al.* (1988) did the first MRI volumetric study of the ventricular system to confirm the CT finding of lateral ventriculomegaly in schizo-phrenia. Rossi *et al.* (1988) reported similar findings. Our laboratory has recently studied 15 pairs of monozygotic twins discordant for schizophrenia (Suddath *et al.*, 1990). This population demonstrated significant ventricular enlargement in the ill twins when compared with the health twins and, again, the affected twin had larger ventricles than the unaffected twin in almost every pair. It is important to note that this finding of relative ven-triculomegaly in ill twins (compared to a healthy genetic match) suggests that even schizophrenic patients without obvious structural abnormality on an MRI scan nonetheless have some cerebral anatomical pathology.

Imaging at first onset

If the neurodevelopmental model of schizophrenia is correct, i.e. if the morphological findings present in adult schizophrenics exist early in life, they must certainly be present at the onset of the illness. While a number of investigators have reported that ventriculomegaly is not a result of either somatic treatments such ECT or neuroleptic therapy, or of length of hospitalization itself (see review by Shelton & Weinberger, 1986), the question that remains is whether the structural abnormalities associated with schizophrenia predate the symptoms. One approach to this question has been the study of recently disgnosed patients. Weinberger *et al.* (1982) looked retrospectively at CT scans done on acutely psychotic patients, most of which were done routinely for diagnostic evaluation. The mean ventricle–brain ratio – a measure of ventricular size – of the 35 first-break patients with schizophreniform disorder (mean age twenty-one) did not differ significantly from that of 17 with chronic schizophrenia (mean age twenty-eight), while both groups differed significantly from a neurologic control group and a control group of patients with other psychiatric disorders. To quote from that paper, '... it is likely that the finding predates the acute illness, probably by a period of years.' Nybäck *et al.* (1982) studied ventricular size in patients with acute psychosis, many of whom were having their first break of schizophrenia. Lateral-ventricular enlargement was reported in the patients, although the authors do not clearly differentiate patients with a definite diagnosis and a first onset of illness from other patients.

The next year, Schulz *et al.* (1983) reported on ventricle–brain ratio measurements from 15 teenagers with schizophrenia or schizophreniform disorder (mean 16.5 years), 8 borderline adolescents, and 18 controls of similar age (scans chosen from a film library). The schizophrenia group, although only ill for an average of 13 months and having received, on average, less than 6 months of neuroleptic treatment, had significantly enlarged ventricles when compared with both other groups. Ventricular size did not correlate with duration of illness.

Turner, Toone and Brett-Jones (1986) prospectively recruited patients with schizophrenia who were within two years of presentation, and compared their CT scans with an age-matched control group of hospital employee volunteers. Ventricle–brain ratios of patients were significantly larger than the control mean.

A multidimensional method of determining which patients have CT scan abnormalities was used by Gattaz *et al.* (1988), in a study of 30 schizophrenics and 30 age-matched controls. They noted that 5 of the 13 patients with deviant CT parameters were first-onset. Iacono *et al.* (1988) compared first-break psychotic patients (31 schizophrenic, 20 schizophreniform, 18 bipolar, and 16 major depressive) with both medical controls and normal controls. The mean age for most groups was approximately 23. These investigators did not report differences between any patient group and either control group for ventricle–brain ratio or sulcal dilatation, although patients with schizo-phrenia had significantly enlarged third-ventricular width when compared with the normals or with medical controls. It is of note that groups were not sex-matched.

Lieberman and colleagues, at Hillside Hospital, New York, are conducting a prospective study of first-break schizophreniform patients (personal communication). Over one-third of the first 60 patients to enter the study, the majority of whom were neuroleptic naïve, show evidence of brain pathology on MRI, including enlarged ventricles. Computerized image analysis additionally shows significantly enlarged temporal horns and smaller hippo-campi in the patients, compared with controls, results which are similar to those of our studies of discordant monozygous twins. Lieberman's group has also noted that evidence of structural brain abnormality correlates with markedly slower subsequent treatment response.

In a recent report, Woody *et al.* (1987) described lateral-, third- and fourth-ventricle enlargement in a 10-year-old with recent onset of DSM-III schizophrenia. The CT was done within two months of onset of psychosis, and MRI confirmed the findings. Scans were repeated four and ten months later, with no change in ventricular size. Weinberger (1988) has since reported the case of a 17-year-old male with newly diagnosed schizophrenia who had received a CT scan fifteen months prior to admission (and before symptom onset) for a sports-related injury. The scan, which showed ventriculomegaly and prominent cortical markings, was virtually identical to a repeat study after admission.

Thus, research overwhelmingly supports the first prediction that we proposed on the basis of a neurodevelopmental model of this illness, i.e. that evidence of neuropathology is not only present during the course of illness, but is present at, and probably before, its start.

Length of illness

The second prediction runs counter to the traditional dementia praecox view of schizophrenia which assumes progressive brain deterioration over time. From the earliest CT studies, there was reason to question this view. It had been previously assumed, based on models of other adult-onset neuropsychiatric illnesses such as Alzheimer's disease and Huntington's chorea, that any pathology in schizophrenia would be progressive in nature, following what was usually thought to be a progressive clinical course. While clinical work has recently begun again to question the latter assumption (Harding *et al.*, 1987), our first CT study (Weinberger *et al.*, 1979) presented results that questioned the former. The degree of ventriculomegaly found in that group of 58 chronic schizophrenics did not correlate with age, length of illness, or length of hospitalization, all surprising findings at the time. If the pathology were progressive, it should have been more apparent in patients who had been ill longer. Even the subtle degenerative changes associated with normal aging produce progressive enlargement in ventricular size. The lack of such change in schizophrenia suggested that the underlying pathological condition was static.

Most subsequent studies that have addressed this question have also failed to find a correlation between lateral-ventricular size and length of illness (Golden *et al.*, 1980; Nasrallah *et al.*, 1983; Nybäck *et al.*, 1982; Pearlson *et al.*, 1985; Schulz *et al.*, 1983; Weinberger *et al.*, 1979; Williams *et al.*, 1985). A recent report by our laboratory, with a new sample of 71 patients, again reported no correlation between CT measures and age at onset, duration of illness, or number of previous hospitalizations (Shelton et al., 1988). Pfefferbaum et al. (1988) used a semi-automated computerized technique to measure ventricular and sulcal volumes of 45 schizophrenics and 57 controls. The controls showed a significant effect of aging on the size of ventricles and sulci. When patients' measurements were corrected for this age factor, significant differences were still found between schizophrenics and controls in all areas. Age of onset and duration of illness again did not correlate with the CT measures.

In studies utilizing MRI, similar results have emerged. Neither Kelsoe et al. (1988) nor Rossi et al. (1988) found a correlation between ventriculomegaly on MRI and length of illness. The ongoing twin study being done by our laboratory (Suddath et al., 1990) again showed no correlation between this finding and length of illness. Thus, research overwhelmingly supports the second prediction made, in that the evidence for pathological changes does not become more apparent as the illness advances.

Premorbid functioning

One could hypothesize that, while many schizophrenic patients have premorbid histories that fall within the normal range, if the neuropathological changes predate the onset of psychosis then this may, nonetheless, be associated with relative, perhaps subtle, premorbid dysfunction. Several studies have looked at the premorbid functioning of patients with schizophrenia in relationship to the presence of structural brain abnormalities.

Weinberger et al. (1980) combined elements from a number of retrospective premorbid assessment scales to collect data on a number of age periods. Patients with enlarged ventricles had significantly poorer premorbid childhood functioning than did other patients with schizophrenia. If sulcal abnormalities were also included, poor functioning was also noted in early and late adolescence for these patients. Takahashi et al. (1981) noted an association between lower educational background and overall CT-scan abnormality in schizophrenia. DeLisi et al. (1983), in a follow up study of 35 schizophreniform patients from an earlier study (Weinberger et al., 1982), found the 7 patients with ventricular enlargement to have demonstrated significantly poorer premorbid social adjustment than the other patients. Williams et al. (1985) found an association between premorbid schizoid traits and ventricle–brain ratio. Pearlson et al. (1985) combined information on the presence of premorbid schizoid personality, poor grade school functioning, and failure to graduate from high school for each of their 19 schizophrenic subjects. The patients with enlarged ventricle–brain ratios had significantly poorer premorbid histories, using this assessment method.

These findings suggest that the structural substrate linked with schizophrenia may be related to, if not responsible for, dysfunctional symptoms that long predate the onset of psychosis. They are also consistent with the view that the neuropathological condition exists early in life. To quote our first study of premorbid functioning: 'The relationship of poor premorbid adjustment to CT scan abnormalities . . . suggests that in such patients a neuropathological process that predisposes to or eventually causes schizophrenia in late adolescence occurs or begins early in development' (Weinberger et al., 1980.)

Longitudinal studies

A second technique used to study possible progression of cerebral pathology in schizophrenia has been the use of repeat scans on ill individuals.

Nasrallah et al. (1986) rescanned 11 male schizophrenics, three years after initial study, at a mean age of 30.5 years. The change over time in ventricle–brain ratio ranged from a 35% decrease to a 115% increase, with no difference in the mean group ventricle–brain ratio. Problems with the study, however, included the small sample size and the use of different scanners for the two phases, making it impossible to evaluate whether changes were related to anything other than methodological variability. In a more recent study by our group, Illowsky et al. (1988) examined 15 schizophrenic participants of an earlier CT study (Weinberger et al., 1979) with repeat scans on the same model machine, seven to nine years later. This study also failed to find progression of ventricular enlargement or of sulcal dilatation. Agreeing with these results was a study by Vita et al. (1988), in which 17 patients had repeat CT scans on the same scanner between 2 and 5 years after the original study (with a mean age at initial study of 26.3 years). The mean ventricle–brain ratio did not change significantly over time, and individual ventricle–brain ratios were found to be highly stable.

It is interesting to note that these results were anticipated in 1962 by Haug, who found no progression of 'atrophy' findings in 20 of 24 patients restudied a mean of 2.5 years after initial pneumoencephalography. Storey (1966) reported the case of a woman who underwent pneumoencephalography at the start of her schizophrenic illness, and again 3.5 years later, with no change seen.

Most available evidence thus suggests that the neuropathology demonstrated by findings such as ventriculomegaly in these patients is present early in the course of illness and is not progressive. This lack of progression suggests that, while the pathology may be necessary for an individual to become symptomatic, it does not alone explain the course of schizophrenia.

Genetics and the role of perinatal insult

As a result of family, twin and adoption studies, it is generally accepted that a genetic factor contributes to the liability to develop schizophrenia (Kendler, 1987). Several groups of investigators have explored whether the genetic liability relates to the structural pathological process linked to increased cerebral-ventricular size. The results have been inconsistent from one study to another. Weinberger et al. (1981), in a study of sibling groups, found no greater likelihood of a positive family history of schizophrenia in patients with large ventricles as compared with patients with smaller ventricles. Nasrallah et al. (1983) compared patients with schizophrenia whose ventricular size was greater than two standard deviations above the study control mean with those patients whose ventricular size was smaller than two standard deviations above the mean. While several factors differed between the two groups, the only significant findings were greater age (32.6 years v. 28.2) and a higher frequency of schizophrenia in family members (32% v. 6%) in the 19 patients with high ventricle–brain ratios. Reveley, Reveley & Murray (1983) used monozygotic twin pairs concordant or discordant for schizophrenia to test the genetic hypothesis. The 7 index cases with positive family histories had significantly smaller total ventricular volumes than the 14 patients without such histories. Moreover, while there was no history of birth complications in the positive-family-history group, 6 of the other 14 had such reported, suggesting to these authors that, in the absence of genetic predisposition, an environmental insult can lead to the illness. While Nybäck et al. (1984) and Pearlson et al. (1985) did not find that family history correlated with ventricular size, Turner et al. (1986) did find a negative correlation between these two variables. Kemali et al. (1987) reported positive family histories in 5 of 37 schizophrenics with normal ventricles and only 1 of 13 patients with ventriculomegaly, although this did not reach statistical significance. Silverton et al. (1988b), working with Mednick and Schulsinger's prospective cohort of children of schizophrenic mothers, looked at the contributions of low birth weight and 'super-high risk' (schizophrenic mother and schizophrenia-spectrum father) toward ventriculomegaly. Birth weight was found to account for 22% of variance in ventricle–brain ratio in the high-risk patients (schizophrenic mother only), but 64% of the variance in the super-high-risk group, suggesting that, in this cohort, genetic loading and perinatal factors interact in determining ventricular size. In another approach to this cohort, Cannon, Mednick & Parnas

(1989), looking at the relationship between six CT measurements and genetic risk (i.e. the 'super-high-risk' group noted above), found genetic loading to be associated with evidence of diffuse cortical and cerebellar abnormalities. Taken together, these studies provide inconsistent data about the relationship between genetic loading and morphological brain changes. The twin study from our group suggests that the genetic issue is extraneous in that affected twins consistently have larger ventricles and smaller hippocampi whether they have a family history of schizophrenia or not. Another problem with the genetic risk studies is worth noting. In most of the studies, genetic loading has been determined by whether or not a patient has a relative with schizophrenia. This approach does not take into account the frequency of illness, which is the critical issue. If one patient has twenty living relatives, one of whom has schizophrenia, and another patient has two relatives, neither of whom has schizophrenia, it is incorrect to label the latter patient as not having a genetic diathesis to the illness.

A history of obstetrical and perinatal complications has for decades been linked to schizophrenia in adult life. Because of the data implicating an early developmental process as the cause of ventricular enlargement, it is logical to wonder whether perinatal complications are responsible for, or result from, this early developmental process. Silverton, Mednick & Harrington (1988a) recently reviewed some of this work. Reveley, Reveley & Murray (1984) found a significant association between birth complications and ventricular size in control twins, but no such correlation in schizophrenic twins who lacked a family history of psychiatric illness. Their results are curious, however, because the positive-family-history twins had fewer birth complications than the normal twins, suggesting the improbable conclusion that a family history of schizophrenia protects against obstetrical complications! Schulsinger et al. (1984) found birth weight to correlate inversely with ventricle–brain ratio in 27 offspring of schizophrenic mothers, including healthy, schizophrenic, and 'borderline' subjects. Pearlson et al. (1985) looked at family, perinatal, and other clinical factors as related to ventricular size in schizophrenics, bipolar patients, and controls. The four schizophrenics with perinatal abnormalities had a significantly increased mean ventricle–brain ratio, as well as increased negative symptoms scores and earlier age of onset. Total brain area did not differentiate the two groups. Turner et al. (1986), comparing 30 DSM-III schizophrenics with 26 age-matched controls, found a significant correlation between 'early physical trauma' (based on family interview regarding perinatal history) and ventricle–brain ratio. DeLisi et al. (1986) reported similar findings. In their study of sibships with at least one schizophrenic member, either birth complication ($n = 4$) or history of head injury was present in seven of the eight schizophrenics with the largest frontal-horn ventricle–brain ratios. Kemali et *al.* (1987) found few perinatal complications in schizophrenics with or without ventriculomegaly. A recent paper by Owen, Lewis & Murray (1988) again addresses this issue with the retrospective study of 61 patients. History of obstetrical complications was obtained from chart reviews. While only a trend existed for a correlation between perinatal problems and increased ventricle–brain ratio, there was a significant interaction between sulcal enlargement and obstetrical complications. DeLisi, Dauphinais & Gershon (1988) did not find a history of 'birth complications' (ranging from gestational bleeding to infections at age 11 months) to predict temporal lobe size in schizophrenics on MRI. Pearlson *et al.* (1989), in a study of 50 schizophrenic outpatients, found a history of abnormal delivery to be significantly associated with enlarged ventricle–brain ratio. Cannon *et al.* (1989) looked at the relationship between six CT measurements and genetic risk or pregnancy and delivery complications. They found their results to support a hypothesis that genetic loading is associated with evidence of diffuse cortical and cerebellar abnormalities, while the combination of high genetic risk and perinatal complications is associated with ventricular enlargement. However, cortical and cerebellar sulcal dilatation has not been observed in any of the studies of first-break patients, a fact which is difficult to reconcile with their hypothesis that the cortical changes predate the onset of the illness.

Taken together, these reports tend to support the notion that obstetrical complications are associated with more obvious CNS pathology in adult patients. Several caveats should be noted, however. The definition of obstetrical complications varies considerably from one study to another. Moreover, retrospective histories of this type are problematic, and it is not inconceivable that families having more-severely ill members, i.e. those who tend to have larger ventricles, may be the most prone to distort in an adverse direction their recollection of birth history. Finally, while it is usually assumed that the obstetrical complications cause the pathology, another explanation may be more correct. That is, the obstetrical complications themselves may be the result of prenatal CNS maldevelopment. This scenario, first proposed by Freud in 1897 as an explanation for the relationship of obstetrical complications to cerebral palsy (Freud, 1968), is increasingly considered as the likely cause of most non-mechanical ostetrical complications (Paneth, 1986).

Anatomical localization and the neurodevelopmental model

At the beginning of this chapter we cited two essential components of a neurodevelopmental model of schizophrenia, i.e. that the causative pathology occurs and arrests early in development, and that ontogenic patterns of the maturing brain are related to the clinical course. Thus, a critical feature of this model is that the pathology be relatively silent or result in subtle problems in childhood, yet result in schizophrenic symptomatology in the finally mature adult. The site of this pathology would presumably be a brain area in which dysfunction can be compensated for in childhood, but not compensated for in adulthood. This is, in fact, an unusual clinical pattern for most congenital brain insults, which tend to be more disabling nearer to the time of occurrence of the insult and less disabling as time passes.

While there are, currently, increasing data from both neuroimaging (DeLisi *et al.*, 1988; Suddath *et al.*, 1989) and post-mortem studies (see Chapter 8 and Kirch & Weinberger, 1986) to localize the pathological process in schizophrenia to the anteriomedial temporal lobes, it would be difficult to reconcile a lesion confined to this area with our model. Primate data indicate that medial temporal lesions are not silent in childhood, and that such lesions tend to result in a temporal pattern of pathology opposite to that seen in schizophrenia, i.e. significant symptoms in childhood that may show amelioration with time (Mahut & Moss, 1986). One caveat should be noted here. The primate data involve gross ablative lesions and their impact on memory. The developmental implications of very subtle lesions that involve non-memory functions of the temporal lobe are not known.

In contrast to lesions of the anteromedial temporal area are those of the dorsolateral prefrontal cortex, an area of brain which does not reach functional maturity until adulthood (reviewed by Fuster, 1989). Damage to this area in young rodents and primates does not produce the same problems with delay tasks and other behaviors that are seen in adult animals (Alexander & Goldman, 1978; Kolb & Nonneman, 1976). Moreover, the pattern of deficit following perinatal lesions to this region is consistent with our model, i.e. is inapparent during childhood and may become clinically significant during early adult life (Goldman, 1971; Tucker & Kling, 1967). Dysfunction of the dorsolateral prefrontal cortex has been observed in physiological imaging studies of patients with schizophrenia (Weinberger, Berman & Zec, 1986; Weinberger & Berman, 1988).

Perhaps the importance of the anteromedial temporal lobe in this illness is not as the site of primary pathology (which it may be), but is rather due to the impact this pathology has on the functioning of the dorsolateral prefrontal cortex. The presence of direct and indirect projections from the amygdala and hippocampus to the prefrontal cortex has been well established, and some temporal-lobe lesions have been found to produce impairment in prefrontal cortical functioning (Fuster, 1989). Preliminary twin-study data from our laboratory give interesting support for a functional interconnection between temporal-lobe and frontal-lobe pathology. In the ill co-twins, the degree of apparent hippocampal pathology on MRI inversely predicts the degree of activation of the dorsolateral prefrontal cortex with the Wisconsin Card Sort task, using regional cerebral blood flow. During this task, which 'stresses' the dorsolateral prefrontal cortex, patients with schizophrenia typically perform poorly and do not show the increase in cortical blood flow that normal individuals demonstrate (Weinberger *et al.*, 1986). Thus, there is interesting experimental evidence supporting the functional temporal–prefrontal link which would make the findings of pathological and neuro-imaging work on the anteromedial temporal lobe consistent with a neurode-velopmental approach to schizophrenia.

Summary

The data that we have reviewed, primarily from neuroimaging studies of schizophrenia, support the conjecture that the 'lesion' of schizophrenia predates the symptomatic onset, and may even be present early in the course of neurodevelopment. We have noted studies that support the site of such neuropathology as involving the anteromedial temporal lobes. If the lesion is an early one, then this fact must be reconciled with the typical course of schizophrenia, i.e. onset of psychotic symptoms only in adolescence or early adulthood. We speculate that the critical 'lesion' is one of the connectivity between temporal–limbic structures and dorsolateral prefrontal cortex, as the latter is notable for its relatively late functional maturity and the relative silence of early lesions. If this is the case, the normal progression of brain development may explain the adult onset of the illness.

References

Alexander, G. E. & Goldman, P. S. (1978). Functional development of the dorsolateral prefrontal cortex: an analysis utilizing reversible cryogenic depression. *Brain Research*, **143**, 233–49.

Andreasen, N. C. (1988). Brain imaging: applications in psychiatry. *Science*, **239**, 1381–8.

Andreasen, N. C., Olsen, S. A., Dennert, J. W. & Smith, M. R. (1982). Ventricular enlargement in schizophrenia: relationship to positive and negative symptoms. *American Journal of Psychiatry*, **139**, 297–302.

Cannon, T. D., Mednick, S. A. & Parnas, J. (1989). Genetic and perinatal determinants of structural brain deficits in schizophrenia. *Archives of General Psychiatry*, **46**, 883–9.

DeLisi, L. E., Dauphinais, I. D. & Gershon, E. S. (1988). Perinatal complications and reduced size of brain limbic structures in familial schizophrenia. *Schizophrenia Bulletin*, **14**, 185–91.

DeLisi, L. E., Goldin, L. R., Hamovit, J. R., Maxwell, M. E., Kurtz, D. & Gershon, E. S. (1986). A family study of the association of increased ventricular size with schizophrenia. *Archives of General Psychiatry*, **43**, 148–53.

DeLisi, L. E., Schwartz, C. C., Targum, S. D., Byrnes, S. M., Cannon-Spoor, E., Weinberger, D. R. & Wyatt, R. J. (1983). Ventricular brain enlargement and outcome of acute schizophreniform disorder. *Psychiatry Research*, **9**, 169–71.

Freud, S. (1968). *Infantile Cerebral Paralysis*, (p. 142). (L. A. Russin, translator). Coral Gables, Florida: University of Miami Press.

Fuster, J. M. (1989). *The Prefrontal Cortex*. New York: Raven Press.

Gattaz, W. F., Rost, W., Kohlmeyer, K., Bauer, K., Hubner, C. & Gasser, T. (1988). CT scans and neuroleptic response in schizophrenia: a multidimensional approach. *Psychiatry Research*, **26**, 293–303.

Golden, C. J., Moses, J. A., Zelazowski, R., Braber, B., Zatz, L. M., Horvath, T. B. & Berger, P. A. (1980). Cerebral ventricular size and neuropsychological impairment in young chronic schizophrenics. *Archives of General Psychiatry*, **37**, 619–23.

Goldman, P. S. (1971). Functional development of the prefrontal cortex in early life and the problem of neuronal plasticity. *Experimental Neurology*, **32**, 366–87.

Harding, C. M., Brooks, G. W., Ashikaga, T., Strauss, J. S. & Breier, A. (1987). The Vermont longitudinal study of persons with severe mental illness, II: long-term outcome of subjects who retrospectively met DSM-III criteria for schizophrenia. *American Journal of Psychiatry*, **144**, 727–35.

Haug, J. O. (1962). Pneumoencephalographic studies in mental disease. *Acta Psychiatrica Scandinavica*, **38**(suppl.), 11–104.

Iacono, W. G., Smith, G. N., Moreau, M., Beiser, M., Fleming, J. A. E., Lin, T.-Y. & Flak, B. (1988). Ventricular and sulcal size at the onset of psychosis. *American Journal of Psychiatry*, **145**, 820–4.

Illowsky, B. P., Juliano, D. M., Bigelow, L. B. & Weinberger, D. R. (1988). Stability of CT scan findings in schizophrenia: results of an eight year follow-up study. *Journal of Neurology, Neurosurgery and Psychiatry*, **51**, 209–13.

Jaskiw, G. E., Andreasen, N. C. & Weinberger, D. R. (1987). X-ray computed tomography and magnetic resonance imaging in psychiatry. In R. E. Hales & A. I. Frances (Eds.), *Psychiatry Update* (pp. 260–99). Washington: American Psychiatric Press, Inc.

Johnstone, E. C., Crow, T. J., Frith, C. D., Husband, J. & Kreel, L. (1976). Cerebral ventricular size and cognitive impairment in chronic schizophrenia. *Lancet*, **1976-II**, 924–6.

Kelsoe, J. R., Cadet, J. L., Pickar, D. & Weinberger, D. R. (1988). Quantitative neuroanatomy in schizophrenia. *Archives of General Psychiatry*, **45**, 533–41.

Kemali, D., Maj, M., Galderisi, S., Salvati, A., Starace, F., Valente, A. & Pirozzi, R. (1987). Clinical, biological, and neuropsychological features associated with lateral ventricular enlargement in DSM-III schizophrenic disorder. *Psychiatry Research*, **21**, 137–49.

Kendler, K. S. (1987). The genetics of schizophrenia: a current perspective. In H. Y. Meltzer (Ed.), *Psychopharmacology: The Third Generation of Progress* (pp. 705–13). New York: Raven Press.

Kirch, D. G. & Weinberger, D. R. (1986). Anatomical neuropathology in schizophrenia: post-mortem findings. In H. A. Nasrallah & D. R. Weinberger (Eds.), *Handbook of Schizophrenia, Vol. 1: The Neurology of Schizophrenia* (pp. 325–48). Amsterdam: Elsevier.

Kolb, B. & Nonneman, A. J. (1976). Functional development of prefrontal cortex in rats continues into adolescence. *Science*, **193**, 335–6.

Mahut, H. & Moss, M. (1986). The monkey and the sea horse. In R. L. Isaacson & K. H. Pribram (Eds), *The Hippocampus* (Vol. 4, pp. 241–79). New York: Plenum Press.

Nasrallah, H. A., Kuperman, S., Hamra, B. J. & McCalley-Whitters, (1983). Clinical differences between schizophrenic patients with and without large cerebral ventricles. *Journal of Clinical Psychiatry*, **44**, 407–9.

Nasrallah, H. A., Olson, S. C., McCalley-Whitters, M., Chapman, S. & Jacoby, C. G. (1986). Cerebral ventricular enlargement in schizophrenia: a preliminary follow-up study. *Archives of General Psychiatry*, **43**, 157–9.

Nybäck, H., Berggren, B. M., Nyman, H., Sedvall, G. & Wiesel, F. A. (1984). Cerebroventricular volume, cerebrospinal fluid monoamine metabolites, and intellectual performance in schizophrenic patients. In *Catecholamines: Neuropharmacology and Central Nervous System – Therapeutic Aspects* (pp. 161–5). New York: Alan R. Liss, Inc.

Nybäck, H., Wiesel, F. A., Berggren, B. M. & Hindmarsh, T. (1982). Computed tomography of the brain in patients with acute psychosis and in healthy volunteers. *Acta Psychiatrica Scandinavica*, **65**, 403–14.

Owen, M. J., Lewis, S. W. & Murray, R. M. (1988). Obstetric complications and schizophrenia: a computed tomographic study. *Psychological Medicine*, **18**, 331–9.

Paneth, N. (1986). Birth and the origins of cerebral palsy. *New England Journal of Medicine*, **315**, 124–6.

Pearlson, G. D., Garbacz, D. J., Moberg, P. J., Ahn, H. S. & DePaulo, J. R. (1985). Symptomatic, familial, perinatal, and social correlates of computerized axial tomography (CAT) changes in schizophrenics and bipolars. *Journal of Nervous and Mental Diseases*, **173**, 42–50.

Pearlson, G. D., Kim, W. S., Kubos, K. L., Moberg, P. J., Jayaram, G., Bascom, M. J., Chase, G. A., et al. (1989). Ventricle–brain ratio, computed tomography density, and brain area in 50 schizophrenics. *Archives of General Psychiatry*, **46**, 690–7.

Pfefferbaum, A., Zipursky, R. B., Lim, K. O., Zatz, L. M., Stahl, S. M. & Jernigan, T. L. (1988). Computed tomographic evidence for generalized sulcal and ventricular enlargement in schizophrenia. *Archives of General Psychiatry*, **45**, 633–40.

Raz, S., Raz, N., Weinberger, D. R., Boronow, J., Pickar, D., Bigler, E. D. & Turkheimer, E. (1987). Morphological brain abnormalities in schizophrenia determined by computed tomography: a problem of measurement? *Psychiatry Research*, **22**, 91–8.

Reveley, A. M., Reveley, M. A., Clifford, C. A. & Murray, R. M. (1982). Cerebral ventricular size in twins discordant for schizophrenia. *Lancet*, **2**, 540–1.

Reveley, A. M., Reveley, M. A. & Murray, R. M. (1983). Enlargement of cerebral ventricles in schizophrenics is confined to those without known genetic predisposition. *Lancet*, **2**, 525.

Reveley, A. M., Reveley, M. A. & Murray, R. M. (1984). Cerebral ventricular engargement in non-genetic schizophrenia: a controlled twin study. *British Journal of Psychiatry*, **144**, 89–93.

Reveley, M. A. (1985). Ventricular enlargement in schizophrenia: the validity of computerised tomographic findings. *British Journal of Psychiatry*, **147**, 233–40.

Rossi, A., Stratta, P., Gallucci, M., Passariello, R. & Casacchia, M. (1988). Brain morphology in schizophrenia by magnetic resonance imaging (MRI). *Acta Psychiatrica Scandinavica*, **77**, 741–5.

Schulsinger, F., Parnas, J., Petersen, E. T., Schulsinger, H., Teasdale, T. W., Mednick, S. A., Møller, L. & Silverton, L. (1984). Cerebral ventricular size in the offspring of schizophrenic mothers. *Archives of General Psychiatry*, **41**, 602–6.

Schulz, S. C., Koller, M. M., Kishore, P. R., Hamer, R. M., Gehl, J. J. & Friedel, R. O. (1983). Ventricular enlargement in teenage patients with schizophrenia spectrum disorder. *American Journal of Psychiatry*, **140**, 1592–5.

Shelton, R. C., Karson, C. N., Doran, A. R., Pickar, D., Bigelow, L. B. & Weinberger, D. R. (1988). Cerebral structural pathology in schizophrenia: evidence for a selective prefrontal cortical defect. *American Journal of Psychiatry*, **145**, 154–63.

Shelton, R. C. & Weinberger, D. R. (1986). X-ray computerized tomography studies in schizophrenia: a review and synthesis. In H. A. Nasrallah & D. R. Weinberger (Eds.), *Handbook of Schizophrenia, Vol. 1: The Neurology of Schizophrenia* (pp. 207–50). Amsterdam: Elsevier.

Silverton, L., Mednick, S. A. & Harrington, M. E. (1988a). Birthweight, schizophrenia and ventricular enlargement in a high-risk sample. *Psychiatry*, **51**, 272–80.

Silverton, L., Mednick, S. A., Schulsinger, F., Parnas, J. & Harrington, M. E. (1988b). Genetic risk for schizophrenia, birthweight and cerebral ventricular enlargement. *Journal of Abnormal Psychology*, **97**, 496–8.

Storey, P. B. (1966). Lumbar air encephalography in chronic schizophrenia: a controlled experiment. *British Journal of Psychiatry*, **112**, 135–44.

Suddath, R. L., Casanova, M. F., Goldberg, T. E., Daniel, D. G., Kelsoe, J. R. & Weinberger, D. R. (1989). Temporal lobe pathology in schizophrenia: a quantitative magnetic resonance imaging study. *American Journal of Psychiatry*, **146**, 464–72.

Suddath, R. L., Christison, G. W., Torrey, E. F., Casanova, M. F. & Weinberger, D. R. (1990). Anatomical abnormalities in the brains of monozygotic twins discordant for schizophrenia. *New England Journal of Medicine*, **322**, 789–94.

Takahashi, R., Inaba, Y., Inanaga, K., Kato, N., Kumashiro, H., Nishimura, T., Okuma, T. *et al.* (1981). CT scanning and the investigation of schizophrenia. In C. Perris, G. Struwe & B. Jansson (Eds.), *Biological Psychiatry 1981* (pp. 259–68). Amsterdam: Elsevier/North-Holland.

Tucker, T. J. & Kling, A. (1967). Differential effects of early and late lesions of frontal granular cortex in the monkey. *Brain Research*, **5**, 377–89.

Turner, S. W., Toone, B. K. & Brett-Jones, J. R. (1986). Computerized tomographic scan changes in early schizophrenia – preliminary findings. *Psychological Medicine*, **16**, 219–25.

Vita, A., Sacchetti, E., Valvassori, G. & Cazzullo, C. L. (1988). Brain morphology in schizophrenia: a 2- to 5-year CT scan follow-up study. *Acta Psychiatrica Scandinavica*, **78**, 618–21.

Weinberger, D. R. (1987). Implications of normal brain development for the pathogenesis of schizophrenia. *Archives of General Psychiatry*, **44**, 660–9.

(1988). Premorbid neuropathology in schizophrenia. *Lancet*, **2**, 445.

Weinberger, D. R. & Berman, K. F. (1988). Speculation on the meaning of cerebral metabolic hypofrontality in schizophrenia. *Schizophrenia Bulletin*, **14**, 157–68.

Weinberger, D. R., Berman, K. F. & Zec, R. F. (1986). Physiologic dysfunction of dorsolateral prefrontal cortex in schizophrenia: I. Regional blood flow evidence. *Archives of General Psychiatry*, **43**, 114–24.

Weinberger, D. R., Cannon-Spoor, E., Potkin, S. G. & Wyatt, R. J. (1980). Poor premorbid adjustment and CT scan abnormalities in chronic schizophrenia. *American Journal of Psychiatry*, **137**, 1410–13.

Weinberger, D. R., DeLisi, L. E., Neophytides, A. N. & Wyatt, R. J. (1981). Familial aspects of CT scan abnormalities in chronic schizophrenic patients. *Psychiatry Research*, **4**, 65–71.

Weinberger, D. R., DeLisi, L. E., Perman, G. P., Targum, S. & Wyatt, R. J. (1982). Computed tomography in schizophreniform disorder and other acute psychiatric disorders. *Archives of General Psychiatry*, **39**, 778–83.

Weinberger, D. R., Torrey, E. F., Neophytides, A. N. & Wyatt, R. J. (1979). Lateral cerebral ventricular enlargement in chronic schizophrenia. *Archives of General Psychiatry*, **36**, 735–9.

Weinberger, D. R., Wagner, R. L. & Wyatt, R. J. (1983). Neuropathological studies of schizophrenia: a selective review. *Schizophrenia Bulletin*, **9**, 193–212.

Williams, A. O., Reveley, M. A., Kolakowska, T., Ardern, M. & Mandelbrote, B. M. (1985). Schizophrenia with good and poor outcome II: cerebral ventricular size and its clinical significance. *British Journal of Psychiatry*, **146**, 239–46.

Woody, R. C., Bolyard, K., Eisenhauer, G. & Altschuler, L. (1987). CT scan and MRI findings in a child with schizophrenia. *Journal of Child Neurology*, **22**, 105–10.

11

Developmental brain abnormalities on MRI in schizophrenia: the role of genetic and perinatal factors

HENRY A. NASRALLAH, STEVEN B. SCHWARZKOPF,
JEFFREY A. COFFMAN AND STEPHEN C. OLSON

The Ohio State University College of Medicine

Introduction

There exists a substantial body of evidence suggesting that the schizophrenia syndrome is associated with both genetic and environmental factors (Nasrallah, 1986b; Tsuang & Simpson, 1988). The genetic evidence comes from family (Guze *et al.*, 1983), twin (Kendler, 1983) and adoption (Kety, 1983) studies. Evidence of environmental influences comes from studies of prenatal (intrauterine environment: Mednick *et al.*, 1988), neonatal (obstetric complications: McNeil & Kaij, 1978), and postnatal (Wilcox & Nasrallah, 1987) brain insults in schizophrenia, all of which suggest that environmental factors may play a critical role in brain development leading to psychotic brain disorders labeled as schizophrenia, and may be additive to or interactive with genetic factors (Mednick & Silverton, 1988).

Over the past few years, a large body of literature has emerged that points to structural brain changes in schizophrenic patients (Nasrallah & Weinberger, 1986). Within the computed tomography (CT) literature, a few reports have suggested that a large ventricle–brain ratio in schizophrenia is associated with positive family history (Nasrallah *et al.*, 1983; Owens *et al.*, 1985; DeLisi *et al.*, 1985), while several other studies suggest that ventriculomegaly is related to perinatal complications (Reveley, Reveley & Murray, 1984; Turner, Toone & Brett-Jones, 1988; DeLisi *et al.*, 1986; Schulsinger *et al.*, 1984; Murray, Reveley & Lewis, 1988). Some have used this evidence to propose a genetic–sporadic dichotomy as a research strategy in schizophrenia (Lewis *et al.*, 1987).

We previously reported a magnetic resonance imaging (MRI) study of schizophrenia (Andreasen *et al.*, 1986), in which smaller cerebral and cranial midsagittal areas were found in schizophrenic patients compared with controls. We suggested that there may be an early impairment of brain development in schizophrenia. The possible contribution of genetic and/or perinatal factors to smaller brain size was not addressed in that previous report.

We present here MRI studies of structural brain changes in schizophrenia. We tested the hypothesis that, if adverse perinatal complications contribute to disruption of normal brain development, then schizophrenic patients with a history of perinatal complications will have smaller cerebral and cranial measurements compared with schizophrenic patients with no history of perinatal complications. We also hypothesized that certain structural brain changes in schizophrenia may be under genetic control, and that differences would be detected between familial and nonfamilial schizophrenia.

Methods

Sample

Schizophrenic patients living in the community were consecutively admitted to the study after signing informed consent. A structured diagnostic interview was used to document the diagnosis. Inclusion criteria were: (1) males and females aged 20–50 years, with onset of illness before age 45; (2) fulfilment of DSM-III-R criteria for schizophrenia or schizoaffective disorder; and (3) the ability to give informed consent. Exclusion criteria were: (1) serious and or debilitating medical illness including seizure disorder; (2) past history of penetrating head injury or neurosurgery; (3) metallic implants in the body; and (4) past or present history of severe substance abuse.

A control group of male and female volunteer recruits from the community (responding to advertisements), matched for demographic variables, were screened with a structured diagnostic interview to exclude those with major psychopathology.

Family and perinatal history

Family history of schizophrenia was obtained by interviews with the parents or, if not available, another close family member. Perinatal history was obtained through a self-administered questionnaire from the mother and, if not available, from the father or other relatives. The list of perinatal complications and methods was previously published (Schwarzkopf *et al.*, 1989).

The schizophrenic patients were classified as family-history positive (FH +), based on the presence of a first- or second-degree relative who was hospitalized for either schizophrenia or a major affective disorder, or had a completed suicide. Absence of such history was considered as family-history negative (FH −).

With regard to perinatal complications, schizophrenic patients were classified as having perinatal complications (PC +) if they had two or more adverse events (Schwarzkopf *et al.*, 1989), and as not having perinatal complications (PC −) if they had none or only one of those events.

MRI scans

Midsagittal MRI scans (Fig. 11.1) were obtained on a General Electric 1.5 tesla scanner using an inversion recovery pulse sequence (TI = 800 MS, TR = 1500 MS). Eight scans per subject were obtained about the midline with a slice thickness of 3 mm and an interslice distance of 1 mm. The midsagittal slice was selected for demonstration of the smallest corpus callosum image and least inclusion of cerebral white matter. The scans were magnified to normal head size, traced, and the following measurements made with computerized planimetry: (1) cranial area; (2) cerebral area; (3) frontal area (defined as the cerebral cortical area anterior to a line drawn perpendicular to the midpoint of the maximum length of the corpus callosum); (4) cerebellar area; (5) ventricle–brain ratio (defined as the ratio of the area of the midsagittal section through the ventricles, to the cerebral area); and (6) area of the corpus callosum and its quartiles. The reliability of these midsagittal MRI measurements has been described elsewhere (Coffman *et al.*, 1989).

Results

Study 1

In the first study, we compared cranial, cerebral and frontal midsagittal areas in schizophrenic patients who are PC + *v.* PC − and FH + *v.* FH − (Nasrallah *et al.*, 1988; Schwarzkopf *et al.*, 1989). We found no differences between the PC +, PC − and control groups, suggesting that for these brain parameters, perinatal complications may not be of etiological relevance. On the other hand, when the FH + group was compared with the FH − and

218

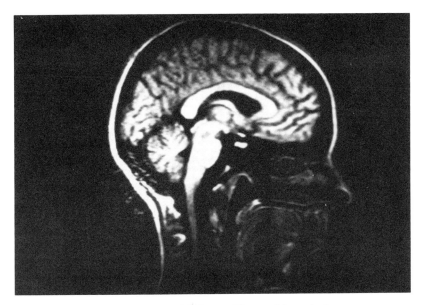

Figure 11.1. Midsagittal MRI scan. The cranial, cerebral,
frontal, ventricular, cerebellar and callosal areas were measured
for each subject on this plane.

control groups, significantly smaller mean brain areas were found in the
FH+ group, suggesting that reduced cranial and cerebral size in schizophrenia is influenced by genetic factors.

Study 2

In the second study, we focussed on the cerebellar vermal lobules. Courchesne *et al.* (1988) reported that, in autism, lobules VI–VIII (superior
posterior vermis) but not lobules I–V (anterior vermis) or VIII–X (inferior
posterior vermis) were selectively hypoplastic, possibly because of adverse
neurodevelopmental events to which lobules VI–VII, but not the others, are
differentially sensitive. We hypothesized that the PC+ schizophrenia group
would have smaller vermal lobules VI–VII than the PC− group but show no
difference in the other lobules.

We found (Nasrallah *et al.*, 1989) that although the total cerebellar area was
not different between the PC+, PC− and control groups, the area of lobules
VI–VII (but not I–V or VIII–X) was significantly smaller in the PC+
compared with the PC− group. It should be noted, however, that the area of

VI–VII was (nonsignificantly) larger in both PC+ and PC− groups, compared with the control group.

The results of this study suggest a role for perinatal complications in the neurodevelopmental dysplasia of the cerebellum in schizophrenia. It is worth noting that we previously reported an association between cerebellar atrophy and third-ventricular enlargement in schizophrenia (Nasrallah *et al.*, 1985). Perinatal hypoxia is known to result in periventricular neuronal death with tissue resorption and subsequent third-ventricular enlargement (Larroche, 1984).

Study 3

In the third study, we examined the possible relationship of perinatal complications to the size of the corpus callosum in schizophrenia. Since the postmortem report of Rosenthal & Bigelow (1972) of increased thickness of the corpus callosum in schizophrenia, several investigators have speculated about the cause of callosal enlargement. In a previous histological study, we found no evidence of change in the number of fibers or glial cells per unit callosal area (Nasrallah *et al.*, 1983). Based on the fact that there is an exuberance of callosal fibers early in neurodevelopment, followed by programmed elimination (Hamburger & Oppenheim, 1982) that continues throughout fetal life, we hypothesized that adverse perinatal complications might interrupt the normal processes of callosal fiber elimination, resulting in the persistence of excessive callosal tissue (Nasrallah, 1989).

We compared the area of the body of the corpus callosum (the middle two quartiles, excluding the genu and splenium) in PC+ and PC− schizophrenia groups. The callosal body was significantly larger in the PC+ group compared with the PC− group, confirming the hypothesis. These findings suggest a role for environmental factors during fetal life for the size of the largest interhemispheric commissure, which may have important impact for the lateralization and psychopathology in schizophrenia (Nasrallah, 1985; Nasrallah, 1986*a*). The importance of controlling for perinatal complications may explain the conflicting literature on callosal dimensions on MRI in schizophrenia (Mathew *et al.*, 1985; Nasrallah *et al.*, 1986*b*).

Discussion

The data of the three studies presented above underscore the importance of both genetic and environmental factors in determining brain structure in adult schizophrenia. Genetic factors appear to be associated with smaller head and brain size in schizophrenia, while environmental brain insults during pregnancy and delivery may result in either hypoplasia, dysplasia or hyperplasia, depending on whether such adverse events interfere with neuronal proliferation, migration or elimination.

There clearly is a need to control for both genetic and environmental events when studying brain anatomy of histopathology in schizophrenia. The evidence is rapidly accumulating that many of the abnormal brain findings in schizophrenia are consistent with neurodevelopmental pathology (Lyon *et al.*, 1989). It is critical that the schizophrenia populations being studied by various investigators for *in-vivo* brain imaging be carefully assessed for both genetic and perinatal parameters. It is quite possible that spurious findings may be encountered if researchers do not control for those parameters.

References

Andreasen, N. C., Nasrallah, H. A., Dunn, V., Olson, S. C., Grove, W. M., Ehrhardt, J. C., Coffman, J. A. & Crosset, J. H. W. (1986). Structural abnormalities in the frontal system in schizophrenia. A magnetic resonance imaging study. *Archives of General Psychiatry*, **43**, 136–44.

Coffman, J. A., Schwarzkopf, S. B., Olson, S. C. & Nasrallah, H. A. (1989). Midsagittal cerebral anatomy by magnetic resonance imaging: The importance of slice position and thickness. *Schizophrenia Research*, **2**, 287–94.

Courchesne, E., Yeung-Courchesne, R., Press, G. A., Hesselink, J. R. & Jernigan, T. L. (1988). Hypoplasia of cerebellar vermal lobules VI and VII in autism. *New England Journal of Medicine*, **318**, 1349–54.

DeLisi, L. E., Goldin, L. R., Hamovit, J. R., *et al.* (1985). Is cerebral ventricular enlargement a genetic marker for schizophrenia? *Psychopharmacology Bulletin*, **21**, 365–7.

DeLisi, L. E., Goldin, L. R., Hamovit, J. R., Maxwell, E., Kurtz, D. & Gershon, E. S. (1986). A family study of the association of increased ventricular size in schizophrenia. *Archives of General Psychiatry*, **43**, 148–52.

Guze, S. B., Cloninger, C. R., Martin, R. L., *et al.* (1983). A follow-up and family study of schizophrenia. *Archives of General Psychiatry*, **40**, 1273–776.

Hamburger, V. & Oppenheim, R. W. (1982). Naturally occurring neuronal cell death in vertebrates. *Neuroscience Commentaries*, **1**, 39–55.

Kendler, K. S. (1983). Twin studies in schizophrenia, a current perspective. *American Journal of Psychiatry*, **140**, 1413–19.

Kety, S. S. (1983). Observations on genetic and environmental influences in the etiology of mental disorders from studies on adoptees and their families. In: S. S. Kety, L. P. Rowland, R. L. Sedman & S. W. Matthyesse (Eds.), *Genetics of Neurological and Psychiatric Disorders* (pp. 105–14). New York: Raven Press.

Larroche, J. C. (1984). Perinatal brain damage. In: J. H. Adams, J. A. N. Corsellis & L. W. Duchen (Eds.), *Greenfield's Neuropathology* (pp. 451–89). New York: Wiley-Medical.

Lewis, S. W., Reveley, A. M., Reveley, M. A., Chitkara, B. & Murray, R. M. (1987). The familial/sporadic distinction as a strategy in schizophrenia research. *British Journal of Psychiatry*, **151**, 306–10.

Lyon, M., Barr, C. E., Cannon, T. D., Mednick, S. A. & Shore, D. (1989). Fetal neural development and schizophrenia. *Schizophrenia Bulletin*, **15**, 149–61.

McNeil, T. F. & Kaij, L. (1978). Obstetric factors in the development of schizophrenia. In: L. C. Wynne, R. L. Cromwell & S. W. Mathyesse (Eds.), *The Nature of Schizophrenia* (pp. 401–29). New York: Wiley.

Mathew, R. J., Partain, C. L., Prakash, R., Kulkarni, M. V., Logan, T. P. & Wilson, W. H. (1985). A study of the septum pellucidum and corpus callosum in schizophrenia with MR imaging. *Acta Psychiatrica Scandinavica*, **72**, 414–21.

Mednick, S. A., Machon, R. A., Huttunen, M. O. & Bonett, D. (1988). Adult schizophrenia following prenatal exposure to an influenza epidemic. *Archives of General Psychiatry*, **45**, 189–92.

Mednick, S. A. & Silverton, L. (1988). High-risk studies of the etiology of schizophrenia. In: M. T. Tsuang & J. C. Simpson (Eds.), *The Handbook of Schizophrenia: Nosology, Epidemiology and Genetics of Schizophrenia* (pp. 543–62). Amsterdam: Elsevier.

Murray, R. M., Reveley, A. M. & Lewis, S. W. (1988). Family history, obstetric complications and cerebral abnormality in schizophrenia. In: M. T. Tsuang & J. C. Simpson (Eds.), *The Handbook of Schizophrenia: Nosology, Epidemiology and Genetics of Schizophrenia* (pp. 563–78). Amsterdam: Elsevier.

Nasrallah, H. A. (1985). The unintegrated right cerebral hemispheric consciousness as alien intruder: A possible mechanism for schneiderian delusions in schizophrenia. *Comprehensive Psychiatry*, **26**, 273–81.

(1986a). Cerebral hemisphere asymmetries and interhemispheric integration in schizophrenia. In H. A. Nasrallah & D. R. Weinberger (Eds.), *The Handbook of Schizophrenia: The Neurology of Schizophrenia* (pp. 157–74). Amsterdam: Elsevier.

(1986b). The differential diagnosis of schizophrenia: Genetic, perinatal, neurologic, pharmacological and psychiatric factors. In H. A. Nasrallah & D. R. Weinberger (Eds.), *The Handbook of Schizophrenia: The Neurology of Schizophrenia* (pp. 49–64). Amsterdam: Elsevier.

(1989). Right-hemispheric speech, callosal size, perinatal brain insult and schizophrenia. *Annals of Neurology*, **26**, 290–1.

Nasrallah, H. A., Kuperman, S., Hamra, B. J. & McCalley-Whitters, M. (1983). Clinical differences between schizophrenic patients with and without large cerebral ventricles. *Journal of Clinical Psychiatry*, **44**, 407–9.

Nasrallah, H. A., Jacoby, C. G., Chapman, S. & McCalley-Whitters, M. (1985). Third ventricular enlargement on CT scans in schizophrenia: Association with cerebellar atrophy. *Biological Psychiatry*, **20**, 443–50.

Nasrallah, H. A., Olson, S. C., Coffman, J. A., Schwarzkopf, S. B., McLaughlin, J. B., Brandt, J. B. & Lynn, M. B. (1988). Magnetic resonance brain imaging, perinatal injury and negative symptoms in schizophrenia. *Schizophrenia Research*, **1**, 171–2.

Nasrallah, H. A., Schwarzkopf, S. B., Coffman, J. A. & Olson, S. C. (1989). Hypoplasia of the cerebellar vermal lobules VI and VII on MRI scans in schizophrenia is associated with perinatal brain insult. *Schizophrenia Research*, **2**, 124.

Nasrallah, H. A. & Weinberger, D. R. (Eds.) (1986). *The Handbook of Schizophrenia: The Neurology of Schizophrenia.* Amsterdam: Elsevier.

Owens, D. G. C., Johnstone, E. C., Crow, T. J., Frith, C. D., Jagoe, J. R. & Kreel, L. (1985). Lateral ventricular size in schizophrenia: Relationship to the disease process and its clinical manifestations. *Psychological Medicine*, **15**, 27–41.

Pearlson, A. D. & Veroff, A. E. (1981). Computerized tomographic scan changes in manic depressive illness. *Lancet*, **2**, 470.

Reveley, A. M., Reveley, M. A. & Murray, R. M. (1984). Cerebral ventricular enlargement in non-genetic schizophrenia: A controlled twin study. *British Journal of Psychiatry*, **144**, 89–92.

Rosenthal, R. & Bigelow, B. (1972). Quantitative brain measurements in chronic schizophrenia. *British Journal of Psychiatry*, **121**, 259–64.

Schulsinger, F., Parnas, J., Petersen, E. T., Schulsinger, H., Teasdale, T. W., Mednick, S. A., Mollder, L. & Silverton, L. (1984). Cerebral ventricular size in the offspring of schizophrenic mothers. *Archives of General Psychiatry*, **41**, 602–5.

Schwarzkopf, S. B., Nasrallah, H. A., Olson, S. C. & Coffman, J. A. (1989). Relationship of perinatal complications and genetic loading in schizophrenia. *Psychiatry Research*, **27**, 233–9.

Tsuang, M. T. & Simpson, J. C. (Eds.) (1988). *The Handbook of Schizophrenia: Nosology, Epidemiology and Genetics in Schizophrenia.* Amsterdam: Elsevier.

Turner, S. W., Toone, B. K. & Brett-Jones, J. R. (1988). Computerized tomographic scan changes in early schizophrenia. *Psychological Medicine*, **16**, 219–24.

Wilcox, J. A. & Nasrallah, H. A. (1987). Childhood head trauma and schizophrenia. *Psychiatry Research*, **10**, 303–6.

Part VI

Conclusion

12

Fetal neural development and adult schizophrenia: an elaboration of the paradigm

TYRONE D. CANNON AND SARNOFF A. MEDNICK

University of Southern California

Introduction

This volume was conceived as an attempt to delineate possible neurodevelopmental processes and mechanisms that may be involved in the etiology and expression of schizophrenia. Our goal was to build bridges of knowledge and theory between several different fields, including developmental neuroscience, obstetrics, neuropathology, psychiatry, and epidemiology. It was hoped that such bridges may help to explain the growing body of evidence pointing to a role of prenatal and perinatal events in the etiology of schizophrenia as well as some of the important clinical-descriptive features of the disorder. In the following paragraphs we assess the viability of this perspective by considering how some of the major etiological and descriptive findings in schizophrenia research may be informed by our current understanding of normal and abnormal processes in fetal neural development.

Neuropathological findings in schizophrenia

A prenatal or perinatal origin of the brain anomalies found in schizophrenics would help to support the hypothesis that the brain abnormalities play an etiological role in the disorder. Four types of neuropathological findings are reviewed in this volume: (1) ectopic changes in the hippocampal formation; (2) density and volume reductions in the limbic system and other regions; (3) ventricular enlargement; and (4) inflammatory or degenerative changes in periventricular structures and other regions.

227

Ectopic changes

Several post-mortem neuropathology studies have found evidence of ectopic changes in the brains of schizophrenics (see Chapter 8). Three findings were most directly linked to a prenatal pathogenesis: (1) disturbances of pyramidal-cell orientation in the anterior and medial portions of the hippocampus (Kovelman & Scheibel, 1984); (2) heterotopic displacement of pre-alpha cell groups in the rostral entorhinal region of the parahippocampal gyrus (Falkai et al., 1988a; Jakob & Beckmann, 1986); and (3) reduced depth of the granule cell layer in the dentate gyrus (McLardy, 1974). These findings imply a disturbance of one or more of three basic processes underlying brain development during gestation: cell proliferation, cell migration, and cell differentiation (see Chapters 2 and 3).

Genetic factors have been linked to ectopic changes in the hippocampal formation of inbred strains of mice (see Chapter 4). Each of these mutations involves either a direct or an indirect disruption of neuronal proliferation and/or migration. Some mutations produce highly specific patterns of ectopia, such as inversion of the laminar organization of the pyramidal cell layer of area CA3c (Hippocampal lamination defect mutation). Other mutations involve considerable variation in phenotype, such as the dreher mutation, in which disturbances of cell proliferation and neuronal migration can affect both the granule cells of the dentate gyrus and the pyramidal cells of the hippocampus. In some mutations the disturbance results in cells which migrate too far; in others, cells do not migrate far enough. These findings are highly suggestive since they demonstrate that genetic factors active during fetal brain development can result in phenotypic structural deviations that closely parallel the ectopic changes observed in the brains of many schizophrenics.

Environmental causes of ectopia and other prenatal disturbances can not be ruled out. The hippocampal formation (and most of the other structures implicated in neuropathology studies of schizophrenics, including the cortex, thalamus, and basal ganglia) undergo prominent cellular migrations in the second trimester of gestation. Areas CA1 and CA2 of the hippocampus are particularly vulnerable at this time (see Chapter 7). The second trimester is also the period when viral infections appear to have a pathogenic role for the subsequent development of schizophrenia (see Chapter 6). Work in fetal sheep has revealed that toxic substances such as viruses can penetrate the developing brain by a number of mechanisms, including receptor-mediated endocytosis, transcytosis, and retrograde axonal transport (see Chapter 5). Steggard et al. (Chapter 5) have proposed that a genetic mechanism may compromise brain-barrier systems in high-risk fetuses. Several autosomal

228

mutations in mice are known to produce immune-system dysfunctions that also have pleiotropic effects on neuronal migration during fetal development (see Chapter 4). In the presence of some form of stress, either a viral infection or substances activated by stress or autoimmune responses in the mother, the normal mechanisms controlling access to the fetal brain could be compromised, resulting in perturbations of developmental processes taking place at that time.

Density and volume reductions

Several post-mortem studies have found reduced cell densities and volumes in various regions, including the cortex (Benes, Davidson & Bird, 1986), limbic system (Benes, 1987; Bogerts, Meertz & Schonfeld-Bausch, 1985; Brown et al., 1986; Colter et al., 1987; Falkai & Bogerts, 1986; Falkai, Bogerts & Rozumek, 1988b), basal ganglia (Bogerts, Hantsch & Herzer, 1983; Bogerts et al., 1985), and thalamus (Dom et al., 1981; Lesch & Bogerts, 1984; Pakkenberg, 1990). While these findings are not as clearly associated with prenatal disturbances, in most of the studies low glial cell counts argued against a recently-active degenerative process. Reduced cell densities and volumes in these regions may reflect a failure of proliferation/migration or excessive neuronal dropout early in life, possibly during fetal or neonatal development (see Chapter 8).

In the case of the hippocampal formation, the same cell groups that are reduced in density have also been found to show heterotopic changes consistent with disruption of proliferation, migration, and/or differentiation during gestation (Falkai et al., 1988a; Jakob & Beckmann, 1986). This observation suggests that: (1) there may be a common source of the two types of anomalies during fetal development (possibly the second trimester); or (2) a primary migratory or positioning disturbance may result in excessive cell death in surrounding tissues via subsequent developmental processes (e.g. lack of development of afferent connectivity, excessive cell elimination).

Ventricular enlargement

Ventricular enlargement is probably the most robust neuropathological finding in schizophrenia. A major issue in evaluating the possible neurodevelopmental significance of ventriculomegaly is the extent to which ventricular enlargement may be correlated with decreased cell densities and volumes in the structures implicated in post-mortem neuropathology studies. Lesch & Bogerts (1984) found that third-ventricle enlargement was accompanied by reduced thickness of the diencephalic periventricular gray matter. Similarly, reduced volumes of limbic structures, particularly the parahippocampal gyrus, appear to be correlated with enlargement of the temporal horns of the lateral ventricles (Brown *et al.*, 1986). In addition, several studies have shown correlations between lateral ventricular enlargement and cerebral volume and/or density deficits on CT and MRI scan (Largen *et al.*, 1984; Pearlson *et al.*, 1989; Reveley, Reveley & Baldy, 1987; Suddath *et al.*, 1989).

The fact that cells targeted for the hippocampal formation and other regions showing volume reductions proliferate in the ventricular zone suggests that ventriculomegaly may be correlated with cell reductions in these regions. In human fetal material, third ventricle enlargement is particularly likely to appear secondary to intraventricular hemorrhage or temporary hydrocephalus during dissolution of germinal matrix at the end of the second trimester; these effects are usually associated with cell loss from the thalamus and upper brainstem at the diencephalic–mesencephalic junction (see Chapter 7). In addition, the geniculate bodies, pulvinar, and ventral posterolateral nucleus of the thalamus are especially vulnerable to birth complications in non-human primates. It is quite possible that disturbances arising during prenatal development interact with or increase the likelihood of disturbances at delivery. Pre-existing disturbances in the ventricular zone (e.g. due to bleeding or increased pressure at the end of the second trimester) could be exacerbated by birth events, the result of which is even greater tissue loss in periventricular regions. This interpretation is supported by a recent CT study in which the interaction of genetic risk for schizophrenia and birth complications was significantly related to the degree of third and lateral ventricular enlargement observed in adulthood (Cannon, Mednick & Parnas, 1989).

It is also notable that the finding of ventricular enlargement on brain scan does not appear to be progressive. In a quantitative review of over 60 brain imaging studies, Cannon (Chapter 9) demonstrated that ventricular enlargement in schizophrenia is not progressive beyond that associated with normal aging processes. Breslin and Weinberger (Chapter 10) reviewed evidence demonstrating that ventricular enlargement occurs early in the course of illness, is not related to duration of illness in a majority of studies, is correlated with poor premorbid adjustment, and shows no significant deterioration in the four longitudinal studies conducted to date.

Inflammatory or degenerative changes

Some studies have found abnormalities that were attributed to degenerative changes. These findings include hippocampal gliosis Nieto & Escobar,

1972; Stevens, 1982), degeneration of the basal nucleus (Averback, 1981), and gliosis of periventricular brainstem and diencephalic structures (Nieto & Escobar, 1972; Fisman, 1975; Stevens, 1982). Gliosis presents a difficulty in interpretation since: (1) gliosis will occur in response to any substantial lesion as early as the second trimester of gestation; (2) the actual numbers of glial cells are high immediately following a lesion but then decline, only remaining high in proportion to number of neurons; and (3) when there is dysplasia of a system, the glial cell counts may still be high in proportion to number of neurons at autopsy (see Chapter 8).

A basic principle in fetal neural development is that processes occurring earlier in gestation can influence processes occuring later (see Chapters 2 and 3). An early insult of cell proliferation, migration, and differentiation could result in a disturbance of developmental processes that extend into childhood and adult life, such as axon detraction and selective cell death. In addition, disturbances in normal afferent connectivities could result in cell death in regions not affected by the initial insult (see Chapter 3). For instance, losses in subcortical cells in the basal ganglia, substantia nigra, and dorsomedial thalamus may gradually be reflected in losses in the prefrontal cortex due to a lack of afferent connectivity. This interpretation is also supported by the fact that white-matter lesions are the most common sequelae of perinatal hypoxia (see Chapter 7).

Thus, an increase in glial-cell counts relative to nerve-cell counts is not inconsistent with a disturbance originating in fetal or neonatal life. In addition, it is possible to have a reactive gliosis that occurs as part of the developmental cascade of events and/or secondary degeneration. At this point, however, we cannot rule out the possibility that degeneration of critical cortical, limbic, striatal, and diencephalic regions originating in adult life is the primary source of the neuropathological abnormalities observed in some cases of schizophrenia.

Regional and temporal specificity

The interpretation of neuropathological studies of schizophrenics is complicated by the fact that the findings do not converge on a single pathogenic process that affects a delimited range of structures. The evidence is more consistent with the involvement of multiple developmental processes affecting many different regions. A neurodevelopmental model is well-suited to explain this heterogeneity since, as we have seen, there is a general tendency for disturbances occurring early in development to cascade and interact with disturbances occurring later. In addition, heterogeneity of phenotypic structural deviations is compatible with the involvement of both single and multiple gene expression. Work in mice demonstrates that cell groups in such disparate regions as the hippocampus and cerebellum can be affected by a common genetic migratory disturbance, and that there may be common gene expression in different phenotypic structural ectopias (see Chapter 4).

Specificity may be achieved by considering processes and regions that are most critical for the expression of schizophrenia within the temporal course of development. Since there does not appear to be a uniform decrease in the size of all brain structures in schizophrenia, it is unlikely that there is a general disruption of cell mitosis over all regions of the ventricular zone germinal matrix. This suggests that disturbances arising in the first trimester of gestation do not play a major role. However, some schizophrenics have been found to evidence a smaller brain size and other gross morphological alterations; these findings could reflect relatively greater expression of the disturbance during the first trimester.

A more likely interpretation is that there are multiple disturbances of cell proliferation, migration, and differentiation during periods and at regions of greatest vulnerability. As noted above, the second trimester is particularly critical for the development of the cortex, limbic system, thalamus, and basal ganglia, since dissolution of the germinal matrix is often a source of hemorrhage and since these structures undergo prominent cellular migrations at this time. These regions remain at increased risk into the third trimester and beyond (see Chapter 7). Within a specific temporal window, genetic or teratogenic effects could produce abnormalities at many actively-developing sites, some of which may not be relevant to schizophrenia, but some of which may be critical in establishing the vulnerability to the disorder. These critical deviations would presumably be those that appear first in development, such as ectopic cells in the hippocampal formation and other regions. Disruptions of subsequent developmental processes affecting cell density and connectivity in both primary and secondary locations may not be required for establishing the vulnerability to schizophrenia but, when present, may make particular syndromal contributions.

Gene–environment interaction

Evidence from twin studies and high-risk studies indicates that neither genetic nor environmental factors are likely to be sole cause of schizophrenia in all cases (see Chapter 6). Most of the evidence reviewed in this volume is consistent with the interpretation that genetic and perinatal factors interact in the prediction of developmental brain changes and later schizophrenia (see Chapters 6, 7 and 9). A basic genetic defect involving prenatal disruption of cellular developmental processes can interact with environmental events arising later in development, such as complications at delivery (e.g. Cannon *et al.*, 1989). However, some schizophrenics do not have an identifiable genetic risk for the disorder. Epidemiological and other evidence suggests that environmental insults occurring during a specific window of gestation can also lead to developmental brain changes and later schizophrenia. It is possible that such effects could mimic the changes associated with genetic factors in cases without a known genetic predisposition. This suggests that there may be replacement of the basic genetic vulnerability to schizophrenia by environmental insults occurring *in utero*.

Latency of onset

The latency between the hypothesized prenatal and perinatal disturbances affecting brain development and the onset of schizophrenia in early adult life poses perhaps the most difficult issue for a neurodevelopmental model of schizophrenia to explain. Several (not mutually exclusive) explanations have been described in this volume: (1) brain maturational factors occurring during late adolescence and early adulthood may result in increased functional expression of developmental brain changes linked to prenatal and perinatal disturbances (see Chapter 10); (2) hormonal changes in late adolescence and early adulthood may interact with prenatal developmental disturbances in the expression of overt behavioral symptomatology (see Chapter 8); and (3) neurodevelopmental structural changes could be critical in establishing the vulnerability to schizophrenia, but stress and other factors arising during postnatal social development could help to trigger the onset of psychotic symptomatology (see Chapters 1, 6 and 9).

It is important to note, however, that the offspring of schizophrenic parents have been found to evidence neuromotor deficits and other behavioral impairments quite early in life (Mednick & Silverton, 1987). In the Copenhagen schizophrenia high-risk project, individuals who later developed schizophrenia with predominantly negative symptoms and schizophrenia with predominantly positive symptoms were found to show premorbid behavioral signs that were analogous to the adult negative and positive symptom complexes (Cannon, Mednick & Parnas, 1990). This work suggests that there is some expression of the underlying neuropathological abnormalities in infancy and childhood. The onset of schizophrenia in cases with prenatal and perinatal structural brain changes is likely to be insidious and difficult to define. In these cases, it may be the lack of ability to perform what is expected as an adult, combined with the stress that this failure brings on, that determines the deterioration in functioning associated with the diagnosis of schizophrenia.

233

Functional expression

If neurodevelopmental brain abnormalities play an etiological role in schizophrenia, then they should be related to important aspects of the clinical presentation of these patients. The brain sites implicated in neuropathological studies of schizophrenics are theoretically very much related to the behavioral and phenomenological features of the disorder (e.g. see Chapter 8). Unfortunately, the empirical evidence bearing on this issue is not very elaborate. There is fairly robust evidence of an association between ventricular enlargement and neuropsychological impairment, but the mechanisms involved remain to be elucidated (see Chapter 9). In addition, preliminary work has found relationships between third ventricle enlargement and reduced electrodermal responsiveness and heart rate activity (see Chapter 9). Another promising line of investigation is the association between subcortical pathology and reduced functional activity in the prefrontal cortex, which could help to explain the lack of initiative, lack of goal-directedness, and apathy that are a prominent feature in many schizophrenic patients (see Chapter 10).

In theory, the heterogeneity of clinical symptomatology in schizophrenia is quite amenable to an explanation based on disturbances of fetal brain development. This heterogeneity could be explained by: (1) the involvement of different brain structures and neurotransmitter systems, depending on the stage of development at which the disturbance occurs; (2) the severity of the disturbance; (3) the extent of secondary degeneration; (4) the involvement of environmental factors during early social development and later life.

Role of neurotransmitters

This volume has not addressed much of the work implicating the role of neurotransmitters in schizophrenia. We regret this shortcoming. One reason for this omission is that not as much is known about developmental changes related to neurotransmitter expression. One important principle was outlined by Jones (Chapter 3), who noted that neurotransmitter levels are closely related to the structural integrity of a system and can change with the development of afferent connectivity and sensory experience. Cells in the striatal–thalamic–cortical dopamine system proliferate and migrate to their target structures in the second trimester, the afferent connections to the prefrontal cortex not being established until after birth. It is possible that disturbances of cell proliferation, migration, and differentiation during gestation influence the expression of dopamine in these cells. It is also of interest that anoxia is known to have subtle but persistent effects on receptor populations (see Chapter 7).

Conclusions

1. Some of the structural deviations observed in schizophrenia are clearly prenatal in origin (e.g., ectopic changes in the hippocampal formation).
2. Phenotypical structural ectopias in mutant mice parallel the ectopic changes observed in schizophrenia in terms of type and location of the cell groups affected and the developmental processes likely to be involved.
3. Prenatal teratogenic factors during the second trimester of gestation may also be responsible for ectopic changes and other structural deviations observed in some cases of schizophrenia. Such effects may mimic the basic genetic disruptions of brain development that create a predisposition to schizophrenia.
4. In many schizophrenics, decreased cell densities in mesolimbic and diencephalic regions (and compensatory ventricular enlargement) are probably prenatal and/or perinatal in origin. We cannot, however, rule out the possibility that some part of the damage occurs postnatally in these schizophrenics or that, in other schizophrenics, most of the damage reflects degenerative changes originating in adult life.
5. The latency between prenatal and perinatal disruptions of brain development and the onset of schizophrenia in early adulthood is a difficult issue. However, the presence of neuromotor deficits and other behavioral difficulties during infancy and childhood in at-risk individuals suggests that there is some degree of expression of the brain anomalies quite early in life. The onset of overt psychosis could be explained by brain maturational factors, hormonal changes, social stress in late adolescence/early adulthood, and other factors.

Acknowledgements

Preparation of this chapter was supported by a National Research Service Award from the National Institute of Mental Health to T. D. Cannon, and a Research Scientist Award from the National Institute of Mental Health to S. A. Mednick.

References

Averback, P. (1981). Lesions of the nucleus ansae peduncularis in neuropsychiatric disease. *Archives of Neurology*, **38**, 230–5.

235

Benes, F. M. (1987). An analysis of the arrangement of neurons in the cingulate cortex of schizophrenic patients. *Archives of General Psychiatry*, **44**, 608–16.

Benes, F. M., Davidson, B. & Bird, E. D. (1986). Quantitative cytoarchitectural studies of the cerebral cortex of schizophrenics. *Archives of General Psychiatry*, **43**, 31–5.

Bogerts, B., Hantsch, J. & Herzer, M. (1983). A morphometric study of the dopamine containing cell groups in the mesencephalon of normals, Parkinson patients and schizophrenics. *Biological Psychiatry*, **18**, 951–60.

Bogerts, B., Meertz, E. & Schonfeld-Bausch, R. (1985). Basal ganglia and limbic system pathology in schizophrenia. *Archives of General Psychiatry*, **42**, 784–91.

Brown, R., Colter, N., Corsellis, J. A. N., Crow, T. J., Frith, C. D., Jagoe, R., Johnstone, E. C. & Marsh, L. (1986). Postmortem evidence of structural brain changes in schizophrenia: Differences in brain weight, temporal horn area and parahippocampal gyrus compared with affective disorder. *Archives of General Psychiatry*, **43**, 36–42.

Cannon, T. D., Mednick, S. A. & Parnas, J. (1989). Genetic and perinatal determinants of structural brain deficits in schizophrenia. *Archives of General Psychiatry*, **46**, 883–9.

(1990). Antecedents of predominantly negative and predominantly positive symptom schizophrenia in a high-risk population. *Archives of General Psychiatry*, **47**, 622–32.

Colter, N., Battal, S., Crow, T. J., Johnstone, E. C., Brown, R. & Bruton, C. (1987). White matter reduction in the parahippocampal gyrus of patients with schizophrenia. *Archives of General Psychiatry*, **44**, 1023.

Dom, R., de Saedeler, J., Bogerts, B. & Hopf, A. (1981). Quantitative cytometric analysis of basal ganglia in catatonic schizophrenics. In: B. Jansson, C. Perris & S. Struwe (Eds.), *Biological Psychiatry, 1981* (pp. 723–6). Amsterdam: Elsevier.

Falkai, P. & Bogerts, B. (1986). Cell loss in the hippocampus in schizophrenics. *European Archives of Psychiatry and Neurological Sciences*, **236**, 154–61.

Falkai, P., Bogerts, B., Roberts, G. W. & Crow, T. J. (1988a). Measurement of the alpha-cell-migration in the entorhinal region: A marker for developmental disturbances in schizophrenia? *Schizophrenia Research*, **1**, 157–8.

Falkai, P., Bogerts, B. & Rozumek, M. (1988b). Cell loss and volume reduction in the entorhinal cortex of schizophrenics. *Biological Psychiatry*, **24**, 515–21.

Fisman, M. (1975). The brain stem in psychosis. *British Journal of Psychiatry*, **126**, 414–22.

Jakob, J. & Beckmann, H. (1986). Prenatal developmental disturbances in the limbic allocortex in schizophrenics. *Journal of Neural Transmission*, **65**, 303–26.

Kovelman, J. A. & Scheibel, A. B. (1984). A neurohistological correlate of schizophrenia. *Biological Psychiatry*, **19**, 1601–21.

Largen, J. W., Smith, R. C., Calderon, M., Baumgartner, R., Lu, R., Schoolar, J. C. & Ravichandran, G. K. (1984). Abnormalities of brain structure and density in schizophrenia. *Biological Psychiatry*, **19**, 991–1013.

Lesch, A. & Bogerts, B. (1984). The diencephalon in schizophrenia: Evidence for reduced thickness of the periventricular grey matter. *European Archives of Psychiatry and Neurological Sciences*, **234**, 212–19.

McLardy, T. (1974). Hippocampal zinc and structural deficit in brains from chronic alcoholics and some schizophrenics. *Journal of Orthomolecular Psychiatry*, **4**(1), 32–6.

Mednick, S. A. & Silverton, L. (1987). High-risk studies of the etiology of schizophrenia. In: M. T. Tsuang & J. C. Simpson (Eds.), *Handbook of schizophrenia, Vol. 3: Nosology, epidemiolgy and genetics* (pp. 543–62). Amsterdam: Elsevier.

Nieto, D. & Escobar, A. (1972). Major psychoses. In: J. Minkler (Ed.), *Pathology of the nervous system* (pp. 2654–65). New York: McGraw-Hill.

Pakkenberg, B. (1990). Pronounced reduction of total nerve cell number in mediodorsal thalamic nucleus and nucleus accumbens in schizophrenics. *Archives of General Psychiatry*, **47**, 1023–8.

Pearlson, G. D., Kim, W. S., Kubos, K. L., Moberg, P. J., Jayaram, G., Bascom, M. J., Chase, G. A., Goldfinger, A. D. & Tune, L. E. (1989). Ventricle–brain ratio, computed tomographic density, and brain area in 50 schizophrenics. *Archives of General Psychiatry*, **46**, 690–7.

Reveley, M. A., Reveley, A. M. & Baldy, R. (1987). Left cerebral hemisphere hypodensity in discordant schizphrenic twins. *Archives of General Psychiatry*, **44**, 625–32.

Stevens, J. R. (1982). Neuropathology of schizophrenia. *Archives of General Psychiatry*, **39**, 1131–9.

Suddath, R. L., Casanova, M. F., Goldberg, T. E., Daniel, D. G., Kelsoe, J. R. & Weinberger, D. R. (1989). Temporal lobe pathology in schizophrenia: A quantitative magnetic resonance imaging study. *American Journal of Psychiatry*, **146**, 464–72.

Index